Other Books by Ruth Sova

AQUATICS: The Complete Reference Guide for Aquatic Fitness Professionals
AQUATICS Study Guide
Aquatics Handbook
Aquatic Exercise
Water Fitness After 40
Painless Strategic Planning
Ai Chi: Flowing Aquatic Energy *(With Jun Konno)*
Ai Chi: Balance, Harmony and Healing
Essential Principles of Aquatic Therapy and Rehabilitation

BackHab

The Water Way to Mobility and Pain Free Living

BACKHAB

The Water Way to

Mobility and Pain Free Living

by Ruth Sova

DSL, Ltd.   Port Washington, WI

DSL, Ltd.
1218 Noridge Trail
Port Washington, WI 53074

Library of Congress Cataloging-in-Publication Data
Sova, Ruth.
    BackHab: The Water Way to Pain Free Living / Ruth Sova
               p.   cm.
    Includes bibliographic references (p. 135)
    ISBN 1-889959-00-6

Revised 2001

Production Editor: Susan A. Harpt, Cheryl Gorton

Copyeditor: Mary Schmit, Gina Taucher

Illustrations: Dave Garacci

Design: InterSection Design, Inc.

Production: DSL, Ltd.

Cover Design: Kurt Sova, Al Esselmann

Printing and Binding: Port Publications, Inc.

Printed in the United States of America   10 9 8 7 6 5 4 3 2 1

DEDICATION

To Mom, Paul, Darlene,

John, Bud, Belle

and all my friends

and relatives

with skittish backs.

In memory of Dad

who taught me

perseverance and sisu.

ACKNOWLEDGEMENTS

This has been a great project because I've learned so much from the people I've worked with on it.

- *Doug McManus, M.D.* trusted me with his patients. He's an incredibly open minded, friendly guy.
- *Lynette Jamison, MOT, OTR/L* reviewed my work from a technical standpoint. She's a warm, caring teacher.
- *Mary Schmit* reviewed it from a logistics standpoint. She has more depth than anyone I know.
- *The Aquatic Exercise Association and the Aquatic Therapy and Rehab Institute* gave me the special training I needed.
- *Angie Nelson, Julie See, Vicki Chossek and Anne Miller* who manage those businesses are wonderfully talented and astute women.
- *Ellen Dybdahl* typed and retyped and retyped. She's an extremely competent and steady friend.
- *My husband, Bud*, helped. He had his back problems at a perfect time in the BackHab project development!
- *Our son-in-law, Dave Garacci* did the illustrations. I love him dearly not only for his willingness to help but also for loving our daughter, Nicole, and making her happy (and hopefully rich!).
- *Our son, Kurt*, did the cover design and photo. He's the best son and friend a Mom could have.
- Special thanks to Mom, Paul, John, Peg, Al, Maria, Jim, and, as always, Kevin.

This has been fun. Working with great people made it that way. I hope the greatness filters through to you.

If you're interested in booking Ruth Sova as a speaker please contact:

Anne Miller Promotions, Inc.
45450 Cottage Row
Chassell, MI 49916

906-482-4333
Fax 906-482-4388
atri@up.net

PREFACE

I hope you enjoy working with the BackHab program. This book isn't about attitude but we all know how important attitude is. Dr. Norman Cousins, who was suffering from an excruciatingly painful disease, found that if he laughed for one hour he was pain free for ten minutes.

We can use the same concept. I believe the water works well for back pain because water is a place for laughing and playing. Approach the BackHab program with a joyful spirit. Enjoy the water. It'll work even better with a playful, fun-loving attitude.

When you're finally pain free, keep smiling and use the preventative program found in Chapter Twelve. Taking time for prevention may be "a pain" but it's nothing like the time you may otherwise take for back pain.

Ruth Sova

FORWARDS

"Ruth Sova has done it again with <u>BackHab</u>! Her writing style is fun and enjoyable and the information is clear and concise. Ruth has a unique approach to pain free living that any professional or consumer can enjoy and learn from. One of her best books!"

Angie Nelson
    -Executive Director, Aquatic Exercise Association, Inc.

"Personal responsibility in wellness is my favorite soapbox and in <u>BackHab</u> Ruth has given the world of 'real folks' a user friendly tool. Her knowledge and practical experience lend credibility to her newest contribution. I will recommend it to the instructors I train and certify and to my class participants and clients."

Mary B. Essert
    - Pioneer aquatic therapy tech, aquatic consultant and educator in Albany, CA

BackHab

The Water Way To Mobility And Pain Free Living

Contents

I. The Background on Backs

II. Treatment

III. Specialization

IV. Prevention

V. Resources

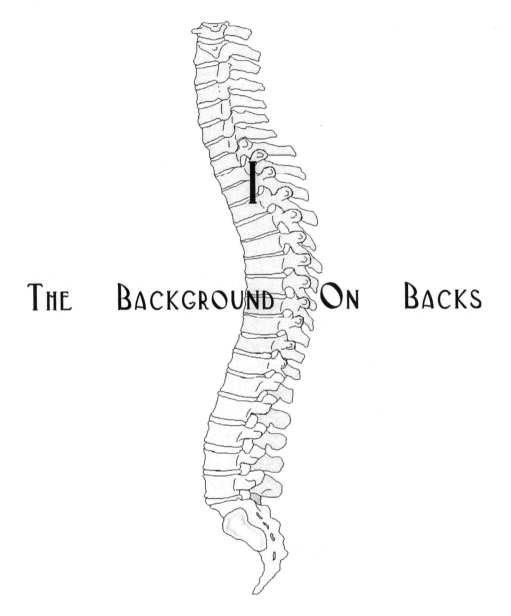

THE   BACKGROUND   ON   BACKS

CHAPTER 1
WHY ME
YOU ARE NOT ALONE

Someone with a bent back who moves slowly and carefully is considered old, yet someone who stands erect and moves with confidence is considered young. It has been mistakenly thought that back problems were mainly a problem for the older adult.

In the United States back pain is actually the most frequent cause of limited activity in persons younger that 45. Doctor D. Imrie in his book Goodbye Backache states that over 30% of the back injuries which occurred in 1979 happened to people under the age of 30. He says, "Back pain is a major - and basically unappreciated - problem for young adults. Although the chronic "problem" backs are seen at a later age, the disease process begins much earlier. The seeds are being sown for the recurring bouts of backache that can make life miserable during our most productive years."

Each of us knows someone, and usually several people, with back problems. The statistics on back pain are astounding:

Although back pain and back problems are almost entirely preventable, they are the number one non-terminal health problem and affect 4 out of 5 adults in this country (Wescott 1992).

Back problems are so commonplace that on any given day in North America 6.8 million people are confined to bed with backache.

It is thought that 80 to 85% of the population will have back problems at some time in their lives (Sova 1991 and LaForge 1990).

While back problems account for 18 million doctor visits a year, approximately 90% of them can be treated at home (Kemper, McIntosh and Roberts 1991).

🐟 *North Americans spend 6 billion dollars per year for tests and treatment for back pain.*

🐟 *Back problems are one of the biggest complaints to account for missed work in the United States. They cause North Americans to lose 200 million workdays per year.*

🐟 *U.S. industry pays 15 billion dollars per year for lost time due to back problems.*

CAN AQUATIC EXERCISE HELP?

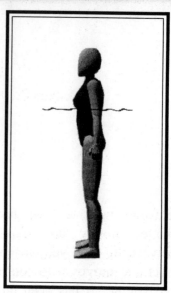

PROPER WATER DEPTH

Because of the relative weightlessness of participants, water exercise is an excellent exercise medium for people who are experiencing some physical difficulty. The buoyant support of the water effectively cancels approximately 90% of the weight of a person submerged to the neck. This means that if you weigh 150 pounds and are neck-deep in the water, you'd only be exercising with 15 pounds!

While the studies on buoyancy were done at neck depth, that is not the ideal depth for aquatic exercise. Midriff depth seems to be best for most people, although a range from waist to armpit is acceptable.

With every footfall on land, the legs and back bear 2 to 5 times the body weight. A participant exercising in water will have very little body weight and very little impact due to the lessened effect of gravity. Since exercisers are protected by the cushioning effect of the water, injuries and stress are far less likely to occur than with land-based exercise. This makes water aerobics the exercise of choice for millions of people who are suffering from back pain. These individuals who are concerned with excess pressure on their backs can safely increase their strength, flexibility and cardiovascular endurance in the pool.

Another wonderful thing about aquatic exercise...since the movements are performed in chest deep water these programs work for the swimmer and non-swimmer alike.

CHAPTER 2
WHY, WHY, WHY?
COMMON CAUSES AND FACTORS BEHIND BACK PROBLEMS

Many factors contribute to the cause of back pain. They include traumatic accidents, stress or tension, poor physical conditioning, osteoporosis, overuse, poor body mechanics, and muscle imbalance. Let's review them quickly.

ACCIDENTS/TRAUMA

Very few cases of back pain involve accidents or traumatic injury. Most injuries that do occur involve lifting a weight of 60 pounds or more. About 75% of these back injuries involve lifting a heavy object from floor to waist level. Unfortunately the people with these injuries are usually in their peak productive years.

STRESS/TENSION

Back pain can also be brought on by stress and tension. We are often unconsciously tense or tight because of stressful situations

in our everyday lives. Stress causes a number of changes in the body as we activate the "flight or fight" mechanism. This stress usually attacks the weakest part

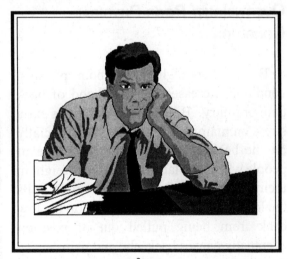

STRESS

of the body. For many of us the weakest part is the back. As the back muscles that are tense or tight get tired of being continually contracted, they notify us by feeling sore, being stiff, aching, or freezing. These muscles that are contracted by tension are being forced to work when no work is required. In other words, the muscles are contracting and working more than normal all day long. This tends to shorten the muscles more, which in turn, causes fatigue, which in turn contributes to more muscular aches, pains or spasms.

Since the muscles in the back are often stiff and weak from imbalance, poor use, or too little exercise, making one wrong move using a tense back can cause a lifetime of low-back pain.

OVERWEIGHT/ POOR PHYSICAL CONDITION

Being overweight or in poor physical condition increases the likelihood of back pain or injury. Being overweight puts extra stress on many body systems but especially on the back. This is particularly true of people who carry large amounts of weight in their bellies or stomachs. The weight pulls the low back forward. The stress on the low back from being pulled out of position eventually causes backache and pain.

Poor physical condition caused by a sedentary lifestyle can also make a person prone to back injury. A lack of regular physical activity lets the back muscles become stretched and weak. After they have become stretched and weak any strenuous

activity may strain and fatigue them. This in turn can lead to muscle spasm or back injury.

A sedentary lifestyle leads not only to a weak back but to weak arms and legs. Lifting that could normally be accomplished by the arms and legs in coordination can't be done. The back muscles become involved and are fatigued by another body part's job.

OSTEOPOROSIS

Osteoporosis is a condition in which the bones become progressively more fragile and likely to cause pain or break. As people

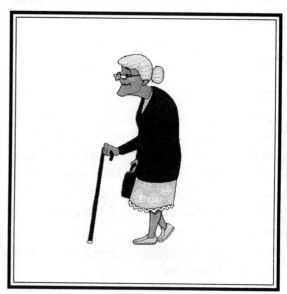

OSTEOPOROSIS

age, bones gradually lose some of the minerals (including calcium) that make them strong. A strong bone is called dense because it's heavy for its size. A weakened bone that has lost some of the minerals it needs is called porous. It's lighter than a dense bone. While a porous bone might be likened to a hard sponge, a dense bone would be like a rock. When the bone becomes porous it becomes weaker and more susceptible to fractures.

Osteoporosis can eventually lead to deformity, disability and severe physical and emotional pain. For more information on osteoporosis see Chapter Nine, "We're All Wet".

OVERUSE

Overusing the muscles in the back is another factor in back pain. Doing too much

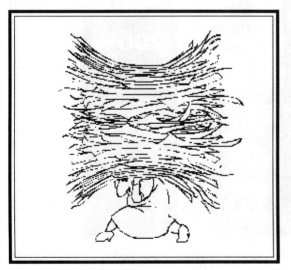

OVERUSE

in one lift or repeated lifts, or in one workday or workout can lead to back strain. Rather than carrying in the groceries one bag at a time, we tend to hurry the process along by carrying too many bags at once. Rather than spreading out the raking, mowing or vacuuming, we try to get it all done in one session. We need to learn to spread out "back" work to whatever we can do without aches or pain.

POOR MECHANICS

Using poor mechanics when involved in Activities of Daily Living (ADL's) is a

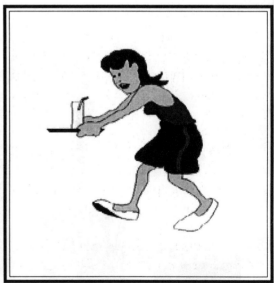

POOR MECHANICS

frequent source of back pain. ADL's include standing, going up and down stairs, reaching, bending, driving, sitting, lying, using long handled tools, participating in sports, lifting, carrying, turning and twisting. How we sit, stand, lie, and move, whether at home, play or work can cause undue "loading" and fatigue.

For example, if your day includes a lot of sitting be sure you're able to sit in a "safe" position. Poor sitting posture causes extra "loading" on the back and will eventually lead to back aches and pain.

"Loading" has to do with the amount of disc pressure on the back during any particular activity. For example, lying down flat on your back involves a lumbar disc pressure of less than 50%. Standing erect with proper posture involves 100 %, sitting erect or standing while hanging forward with arms hanging forward is approximately 150% and standing while hanging forward with arms out to the sides or sitting while leaning forward is approximately 200%. (Imrie 1983, Phillips 1992)

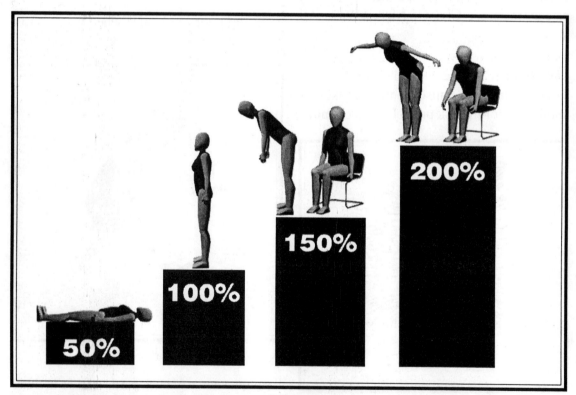

SPINAL LOADING

Obviously, using poor body mechanics while performing ADL's is a key contributing factor in back pain. For more detailed information on proper body mechanics see Chapter Eight, "An Ounce of Prevention."

MUSCLE IMBALANCE

Although all the previously listed factors contribute to back pain, most of the problems (80%) are thought to come from muscle imbalance (Westcott 1992, LaForge 1991). Weak abdominal muscles combined with tight back muscles, and strong hip flexors (muscles in the front of the hip joint) combined with weak hip extenders or gluteals (the muscle behind the hip joint) seem to cause the bulk of back pain in the United States.

Muscles which are subjected to repeated overload adapt by becoming stronger and wider in diameter. Unless they are specifically overloaded with a stretch, they will also become permanently tighter and shorter. When one muscle is consistently strengthened and the opposing muscle ignored, the strengthened muscle will become permanently shortened and the opposing muscle will remain lengthened, weak and inefficient.

Muscle balance is achieved when both muscle groups in a pair are developed to the same degree. Imbalance, resulting from over development or under development of one member of the pair, can cause poor posture, pain, tendon tightness, and eventual misalignment of the body's framework.

Good posture or alignment is necessary for good muscle balance and back health. The back is designed with natural and necessary curves. There are forward curves in the neck and low back, and a backward

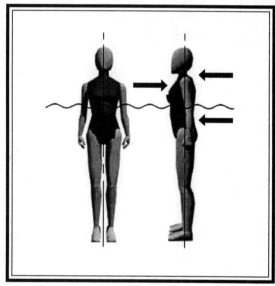

GOOD POSTURAL ALIGNMENT

curve in the upper back. They are *good* curves *if* they're moderate. When these "neutral" curves are decreased or increased there is additional stress put on the spine.

Good postural alignment will allow the

human body to move safely. From a front view, the shoulders should be equally aligned over the hip joints and the pelvis should be resting over the hip joints in a balanced position.

From the side view, the spine should have an anterior curve in the cervical and lumbar areas and a posterior curve in the thoracic area. The ear, shoulder, hip and ankle joints should fall into a plumb line. When deviation from good postural alignment exists in one area, there is always a reactive deviation in another area.

For more information on alignment please see Chapter Six, "Rules, Rules, Rules."

CHAPTER 3

WHAT GOES WHERE

THE WORKINGS AND WORK OF THE BACK

Our backs are made up of three elements: the bones (also called the vertebrae), the discs which are cushions that separate each bone, and the muscles and ligaments (also called connective tissues) which allow movement and hold everything together.

The "spine" or "spinal column" generally refers to the entire package. When people refer to the spine or spinal column they usually mean the bones, the discs and the muscles and ligaments throughout the entire spine. The spinal column has three different functions that it does for the body. It supports the body structurally (helps us stand), it protects the spinal cord (the nerves encased in the spine), and it assists in movement.

THE SPINAL CORD

The spinal cord is a transmission cable that carries the impulses and messages from the brain to all parts of the body. It has nerve roots emerging along each side of it from each vertebra along the spine.

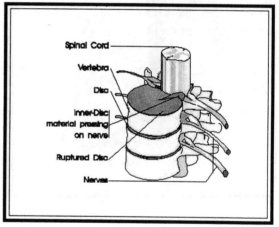

SPINE

DISCS

Between each vertebra is a disc. It is a capsule of jelly-like fluid that acts as a shock absorber for the spine. The disc compresses when weight is put on it, and springs back to its original shape when the weight is removed.

The discs also act as a hydraulic system which disperses pressure on the spine evenly in all directions along the back. Even though the "load" may occur in a particular area, the discs spread it out throughout the spine. If the disc is damaged or bulging, it can exert pressure on the nerve root and cause pain. This is often the origin of back pain.

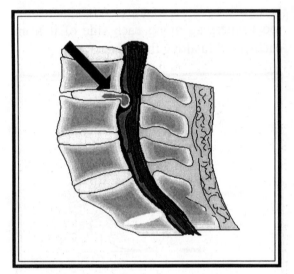

RUPTURED DISC

THE SPINAL COLUMN

The spinal column is made up of five different regions. The cervical spine (neck), the thoracic spine (in the chest area), the lumbar spine (low back), the sacrum (beneath the low back) and the coccyx (the tailbone).

The cervical area of the spine is made up of seven small vertebrae or bones (called C1-7). The "C" means "cervical". The highest vertebrae is C1 and the lowest in the cervical area is C7. The cervical part of the spine is the part that moves when you look sideways, shake your head yes or no, or tilt your ear toward your shoulder. The spinal cord that runs down the center of this part of the spinal column is protected by the cervical vertebrae. It has 8 sets of nerves which carry impulses for motion and sensation to and from the head, shoulders, chest and arms. If you experience ailments in those areas they may be caused by problems in the cervical spine.

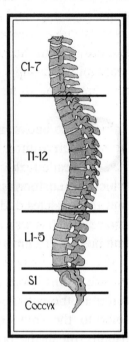

SPINAL COLUMN

The thoracic area of the spine is made up of 12 vertebrae (T1-12), each of which is attached to two ribs. This area of the spine is quite stable and moves very little. Few people have problems in this area.

The lumbar area of the spine is made up of five broad and heavy vertebrae (L1-5). They support much of the weight of the upper body. The nerves that are protected by the lumbar vertebrae carry impulses for motion and sensation to and from the low back, groin, hips, legs and feet. Numbness or pain in one of those areas can often be traced back to a problem in the lumbar spine. This area needs muscular support from the abdominals, back and leg muscles to avoid injury.

In terms of movement, these three areas of the spine have three basic types of moves they can accomplish. They can flex and extend (bend forward and back), they can laterally flex (bend to the side), and they can rotate (twist). This means that both the neck and the waist can bend forward and back (nodding yes or bowing), they can bend to the side (tilting your ear to your shoulder or doing a sidebend), and they can both twist (looking over your shoulder or twisting from the waist). They can also circumduct, but that won't be discussed here.

The sacrum (Sl) is made of five separate bones that are fused together. It is located just below the lumbar area of the spine and is very strong, immobile and fairly immune to injury.

The coccyx is called the tailbone. It is made up of four small bones and is usually injured only in falls.

MUSCLES

The low back (lumbar) and neck (cervical) areas of the spine need good muscle support because they have no stability from the ribs, unlike the chest (thoracic) area. The low back and neck areas rely almost exclusively on muscles to keep them up, stable, or moving. The chest area doesn't need much muscle power because it's connected to the ribs and is supported by them.

There are four groups of muscles that work together to make the lumbar area of the spine function safely. They are 1. the Erector Spinae (back muscles), 2. the Rectus Abdominus (stomach muscles), 3. the

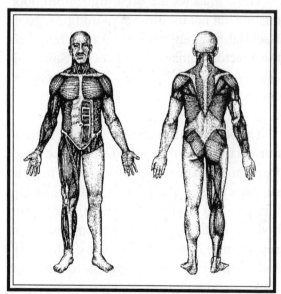

MUSCLES

Obliques and Quadratus Lumborum (midriff or trunk muscles), and 4. the Hip Flexors, Extensors, Adductors and Abductors (the hip joint muscles). If any one of these muscles is weak, or tight (too short), or stretched (too long), or too strong, the spine will not be in proper alignment. This will add wear and tear on the spine and increase the likelihood of back pain and injury.

The **Erector Spinae** are the low back muscles. They hold you up when you bend forward so you don't collapse forward. They also pull you back up when you stand up from leaning forward; for instance, after bending forward or when getting out of a chair.

These muscles are often tight from poor posture but not usually very strong. A good BackHab program will stretch and strengthen the Erector Spinae. The Erector Spinae is usually called the "low back" in the exercise community.

The **Rectus Abdominus** is a long narrow muscle that runs down the front of the torso from the rib cage to the pelvis. This muscle supports the spinal column from the front. In this position it supports one-third of your body weight. The Rectus Abdominus is the supporting muscle on the front of the body and keeps you from hanging forward or back. Although the muscle can be strengthened by exercise, it is usually very weak and not strong enough to do a good support job. Fat in the stomach area stretches the abdominal muscle and keeps it from contracting tightly enough to protect the back.

This muscle is usually very weak and often stretched out. It needs to be strengthened in a BackHab program. It is often call "abs", "abdominals" or "the abdominal muscle".

The **Obliques** and **Quadratus Lumborum** are muscles that lie along the side of the torso. They have a criss-cross pattern that allows them to be very strong and effective. They are responsible for twisting and for bending sideways.

These muscles are usually fairly balanced. They only need controlled use in a BackHab program. They are usually called the trunk, torso or midriff muscles. The Obliques are sometimes grouped with the Abdominals.

The **Hip Flexors**, located in the front of the hip joint, are the muscles that cause the hip to bend (they make your knee come up).

Since they are involved in walking, jogging, kneelifts and kicks, they are quite strong and often shortened from being used so much. They need to be stretched in a BackHab program. They are called Hip Flexors or Iliopsoas.

The **Hip Extensors** are responsible for straightening the leg at the hip. These muscles are found in the buttocks.

The Hip Extensors are usually quite weak and stretched out. They need to be strengthened in a BackHab program. They may be called the butt muscles or the gluts (pronounced like glue) which is short for gluteals.

The **Hip Abductors and Adductors** are responsible for moving the leg sideways away from the body, back to the body, and also across the body. The abductors are located on the outside of the hip and assist in balance. The adductors are located on the inside of the thigh and provide stability for the pelvis.

They both need regular use in a BackHab program. They are usually called Adductors and Abductors.

All these muscles combined with cartilage and connective tissues (tendons and ligaments) support the spinal column. The cartilage acts as a shock absorber. The ligaments and tendons bind all the muscles and bone together. Ligaments attach bone to bone to stabilize them by connecting across the joints. Tendons attach muscles to bones and muscles to muscles. They affect flexibility and range of motion in the joint.

CHAPTER 4

WHAT CONDITION MY CONDITION IS IN

ASSESSMENT AND TESTING

There are several ways to check your back strength and flexibility. Some are simple tests that check only one aspect of back movement but may determine your overall back health. Other tests are complex that check an entire series of movements.

Dr. Hans Kraus and Dr. Sonja Weber have devised a muscle test to determine if people have enough strength and flexibility to handle their weight and height. This test, called the Kraus-Weber Muscle Test, is widely used to assess candidates for low back pain. For those who are interested in the series of 6 test movements, the Kraus-Weber Muscle Test is copied in The Y's Way to a Healthy Back by Alexander Melleby.

The two most common self-assessment testing movements are the toe touch and the situp. These two moves are also the ones most frequently failed by people who have back pain.

If you have been approved by a medical care practioner to do these tests, the procedures follow. If you have not, please discuss them with a health care professional before testing yourself.

THE TOE TOUCH...
Testing the flexibility of the back and back of the thighs.

In a standing position with feet together and knees straight, hang forward. Slowly and gently try to touch your toes with your fingertips. If you can touch your toes, try to touch the floor in front of your toes. Measure the distance from your fingertips to the floor. You should be in an easy, relaxed forward hang during the measuring. Do not strain or bounce. Stop the movement if your back hurts.

If you are unable to touch the floor or your toes you are considered a candidate for back problems. Your hamstring and back muscles

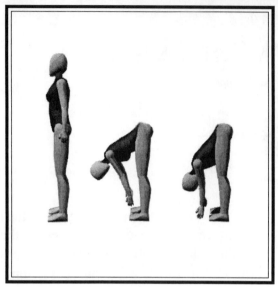

TOE TOUCH

are probably too tight or strong in comparison to the other support muscles.

THE SITUP...

Testing the strength of the stomach and hip flexor muscles.

Lie on your back with your feet flat on the floor and your knees bent as much as possible. Your heels should be close to your body. With someone or something holding your feet down, roll up into a sitting position. Be sure the body (spine) is curling and not straight. Measure the distance between the floor and your shoulders.

If you are unable to roll all the way up into a sitting position you may be a candidate for back problems. Your abdominal muscles are

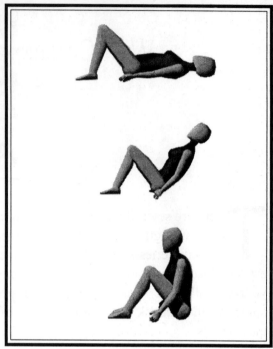

SIT UP

probably too weak in comparison to the other support muscles.

If one or both of these tests can not be accomplished both of these tests can be redone after 8 weeks of Backhab.

It is vital to remember that *these movements are tests, not exercises*. They are not considered wise movements to use during exercise or to try repeatedly. Exercises that will improve the results of the test are listed and described later.

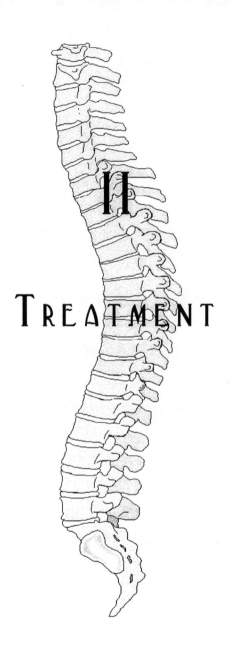

II

TREATMENT

CHAPTER 5

HOMELY ADVICE

HOME TREATMENTS FOR HOME TREATABLE BACK PROBLEMS

Treatments for persons with back pain are as varied as the people who are experiencing the pain. Often, what works for one person will not work for another. Too often, however, the suggested treatments simply cover the symptoms and don't work toward alleviating the source of the problem.

Several different treatments that work toward alleviating the source of the problem can be used at home. Kemper, McIntosh and Roberts (1991) suggest asking yourself these three questions:

 Are there periods of at least ten minutes each day when you have no pain?

 Is all of your pain in the back or above the knee?

 Have you had several episodes of low

back pain over the past months or years?

Kemper, McIntosh and Roberts say that "if you can answer yes to all of them you are an ideal candidate for resolving your back problem on your own".

TREATMENTS

Several of the home-treatment possibilties are listed here.

Weight Control

A sensible weight control program eating well balanced meals can help you control your weight, and often, your back pain. Simply causing less load on the back will often eliminate pain.

Laughter

Many books and videos are on the market showing that injuries, illness and pain can be improved with laughter. The physiological processes that occur in the body during a good belly laugh are beneficial to almost all the systems of the body. Laughter will help to lessen the pain by producing endorphins (natural pain killers in the body) and it will help to lessen the back problem by releasing stress.

Time Management and Stress Management

Taking classes, reading books or watching videos that help you cope with the stressors in your life will often help you with your back problems.

Relearn Activities of Daily Living

Attend classes, read books or watch videos that help you learn how to safely stand, go up and down the stairs, reach, bend, drive, sit, lie, participate in sports, lift, carry, turn, twist, and use long handled tools. Improving your posture and movement patterns can often be all you need to relieveyour back problems. Chapter Eight, "Straight up", has helpful hints to get you started.

Exercise

It has been shown that proper types of movement are more beneficial than bed rest. A study done in Sweden tested people who had regularly missed work due to back pain during the prior year and a half. One half of the group rested in bed each time they missed

work due to back pain during the next year and a half. The other half of the group participated in one hour of exercise (including strengthening and flexibility work) once a week. Over the test year and a half, the exercise group had less back pain and their missed work due to back pain decreased by 50%!

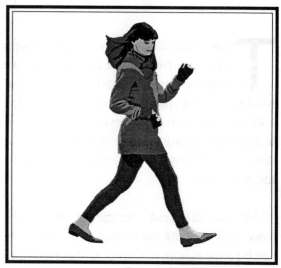

EXERCISE

The Physician and SportsMedicine magazine recommends low impact, conservative exercise. Dr. Schatz in an article called, "Walk Your Back to Health" says that walking is a great aerobic exercise that is safe for people who have had low back injury or surgery. Walking is safe because it is low impact. It helps to relieve pain because it uses the muscles rhythmically and produces endorphins (the body's natural pain relievers). It gives walkers time to think about and improve their posture and alignment. It can help with weight control and improve your mental outlook.

A sedentary lifestyle (or too much bedrest) is linked with all of the following ailments:

Low energy
Arthritis
Obesity
Poor muscular strength and general weakness
Increased stress and tension
Heart conditions
High cholesterol
Constipation
Diabetes
Hypertension or high blood pressure
Osteoporosis
Insomnia
Depression
Increased back problems
Stiffness
Decreased range of motion
Decreased vital capacity
Senility
Pain
High blood sugar

Regular exercise has been shown to have a myriad of benefits some of which are listed here. Exercise can produce these results:

Improve the quality of life
Regulate the blood sugar levels
Control hypertension and blood pressure
Lower the mortality rate
Improve some mental functions
Decrease anger, anxiety and impulsiveness
Improve sexual interest and satisfaction
Increase energy level
Decrease arthritis pain
Maintain a healthy body weight
Improve heart functions
Regulate cholesterol
Improve regularity
Maintain bone density
Maintain healthy sleep patterns
Improve mental outlook
Decrease back pain
Increase flexibility
Increase lung capacity
Lessen overall chronic pain

Following a basic BackHab program can assist you in achieving these benefits.

NON-TREATMENTS

Please note that some back problems cannot be treated at home. If any of the following situations apply, you should call and visit a medical health care professional:

Severe pain that extends below the knee.

Weakness, numbness or tingling in the foot or toes.

Back pain which has followed a recent
accident.

Back pain which is followed by bladder
problems.

Illness in conjunction with back pain.

CHAPTER 6
RULES, RULES, RULES
BACKHAB HINTS, TRICKS, AND GUIDELINES

It's important when exercising to follow certain basic guidelines and precautions. Several that should be adhered to with the BackHab Program are listed here:

Work to the point of tension not pain. Your muscles and body should feel the effort but the effort should not be painful.

The two hour pain rule applies to low back pain participants. If you have more pain two hours after exercising, you probably attempted to do too much during the exercise session.

If you experience pain, stop exercising. Examine the cause, if possible, so that you can eliminate it next time you exercise.

Work toward good muscle balance. Most muscles come in pairs. One of the pairs is usually stronger than the other. We should strengthen and stretch both muscles in the pair but plan to strengthen the weak or stretched muscles more than their stronger, tighter partners. Also stretch the strong or

tight muscles more than their weaker, more stretched out partners. The exercise plans in Chapters Seven and Nine will do that for you.

Use good shoes. Using shoes that are designed for aquatic exercise or aerobics can protect you from impact shock, protect you from slipping, and protect you from rubbing the bottom of your feet raw.

Cushioned shoes will help absorb some of the impact and make the workout kinder to your back. Shoes should also grip the bottom of the pool. That will help alleviate any possibility of slip induced back pain. Slipping on the pool bottom or on the deck can easily reinjure the back. The gripping shoe soles will also help you keep your balance and footing. Adding shoes will also protect you from wearing away an excessive amount of skin from the bottom of your feet.

Choose a good water depth. You should begin in the shallow water. Waist depth would be appropriate. As you begin to get the feel for working in the water you may want to move to deeper water to give yourself more buoyancy and less stress of impact. Finding an adequate water depth can lessen the likelihood of injury. This is usually midriff depth. Be sure the water depth allows you time to move in a controlled manner.

Find a good water temperature. You may need warmer than average water temperature to keep the body core temperature up while doing the very basic workout. You'll probably find 86 to 90F degree water ideal for the workout you're going to do. Water temperature in the 78 to 83F degree range seems to be ideal for people with low back pain who can exercise in regular vigorous aerobic programs.

Stay away from aquatic exercise equipment. Weights, resistance equipment and buoyant equipment should not be used if you have low back pain. The exception is if the equipment is being used to keep you buoyant in the deep end of the pool.

Use good body alignment. The human body is designed for movement and with proper mechanics, it is not likely to break down with use. When the body is in good mechanical alignment, all the forces acting upon it, both internal and external are balanced. When a deviation from good postural alignment exists in one area, there is always a reactive deviation in another area.

Proper body alignment is extremely important in all exercise programs but especially in this one. Alignment simply means posture, or how you're holding your body. Proper posture allows the weight of your body to be balanced. This avoids overworking the back muscles. Here is the proper alignment:

From the front view, if an imaginary line were drawn down the center, the body should be equal on both sides. You will move out of this position for some exercises but it is important to move back into it as soon as the exercise is over.

If a properly aligned body were cut in half down the middle, each side would look equal. The center of the hip joint, the center of the knee and the center of the ankle would all be in a vertical line.

From a side view, the ear should be centered over the shoulders and the shoulders over the hips. *This is an extremely important postural and safety tip*. Leaning forward or letting your head lean forward puts undue stress on the back muscles.

When the body is in proper positioning, it

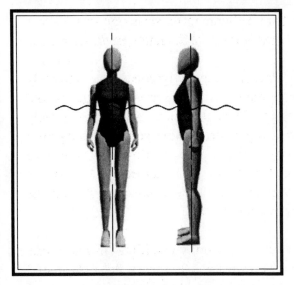

PROPER POSTURAL ALIGNMENT

is said to have an aligned neutral position. This is also called good alignment, proper alignment and good pelvic mechanics.

When body segments are aligned, there is less likelihood of strain in the muscles and ligaments.

Deviations from proper body alignment can be caused by genetic defect or injury, but are more often caused by muscle weakness and imbalance.

Here are some hints to help with maintaining good postural alignment:

Let your shoulders drop away from your ears. Shoulders move up from stress and if the water temperature is a little cool. Relax the shoulders and upper back muscles.

Think about lifting your rib cage.

Think about lifting your pubic bone up toward your navel, but...allow your natural back curves to remain in place. Do not try to move with a completely flat back.

Imagine a helium balloon holding your head up.

Imagine a string coming out of the top of your head lifting the weight of your head for you.

Think about your head moving up, not forward.

If no specific arm movements are listed, allow your arms to move naturally with the exercise.

Move easily and naturally through the water. Only challenge yourself for the specific exercises that ask you to do so. Trying to lengthen your stride during the entire program can cause back stress. You'll usually be able to tell if you're trying to move too far or too fast. You will lean forward.

Keep imagining how you look from the front view and from the side view. Simply imagining yourself standing tall will help keep you in alignment!

CHAPTER 7
FINALLY
THE BACKHAB PROGRAM

C reate your own workout from the choices below. Always begin with the Warmup and Alignment Work and always include the Back Stretching and Abdominal Tightening section either near the beginning or the end of the workout.

When first beginning this workout, spend only 10 to 15 minutes for each exercise session. If you have no pain that you feel is caused or exacerbated (made worse) by the exercises, increase the workout time by about 5 minutes each week.

After easing into the workouts, try to spend at least 15 minutes for each workout. A workout lasting 30 minutes would probably be ideal. Try to work out at least 3 times a week. Naturally, more time and more frequency will help you achieve faster and better results. If, however, you begin to experience pain from the exercises, you'll need to back up and spend less time with each workout. Move forward only when your body is ready for it.

WARMUP AND ALIGNMENT WORK

Begin by walking forward and backwards through the water at hip to midriff depth. Roll from heel to toe going forward and toe to heel going backwards. Continue for 4 minutes. Every 30 seconds mentally visualize yourself in a perfectly upright posture. If viewed from the side, your ear would be directly over your shoulder, your shoulder over your hip and your hip over your ankle. Move slowly until you feel sure that your alignment (upright posture) is perfect. Keep breathing normally.

BACK STRETCHES AND ABDOMINAL TIGHTENING

Now move to the pool edge. This section is for toning and flexibility. Face the pool edge and with your elbows in the gutter, pull both knees to your chest and round your back by leaning forward over your knees (FIGURE1, P. 32). Each time your knees and shoulders move toward each other, think about pressing your navel back toward your spine. Repeat this 6

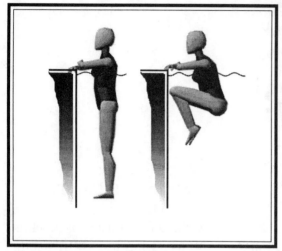

FIGURE 1

times. Stand and rest between each repetition.

Next, stand with buttocks touching the pool wall. Feet should be shoulder width apart and knees should be slightly flexed. Contract the abdominals so the middle of the back presses to the pool wall. This is called a pelvic tilt (FIGURE 2). Hold that position for five

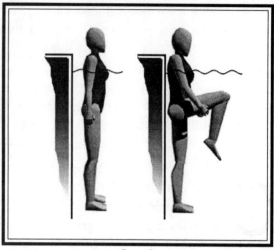

FIGURE 3

seconds and then relax for five seconds. Repeat five to ten times depending on how you feel. If you feel any back strain you should stop and rest and then move on.

Now maintaining an upright torso, pull your right knee up toward your chest and

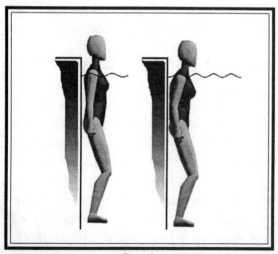

FIGURE 2

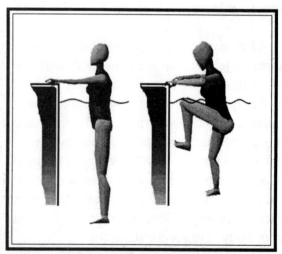

FIGURE 4

hold that position for 10 seconds (FIGURE 3, P.32). Repeat with the left.

Now face the pool edge. With both hands holding the gutter or pool edge, put one foot on the wall of the pool. Tuck your knee and pull your shoulders in toward the pool edge (FIGURE 4, P.32). Hold for 5 seconds. Slightly straighten your knee and arms, round your back and hold for 5 seconds. Repeat these moves 5 times, alternating right and left legs.

ALIGNMENT AND ABDOMINAL WORK

Return to easy walking with the upright posture you began with. Remember to walk forward <u>and backwards</u> (FIGURE 5). After one minute of mentally visualizing the correct alignment, begin to contract the abdominal muscles on every fourth step. Picture a sponge in your stomach. On every fourth step,

squeeze the sponge out with force (FIGURE 6). As you squeeze the sponge, you should breathe out as though something hit you in the stomach. In your head, or outloud, you can repeat "1, 2, 3, squeeze". Walk slowly. When you're comfortable with the cadence, you might help yourself maintain good alignment by switching to, "tall, tall, tall, squeeze". Lift your ribs and stand up tall on the first 3 steps. Pull your stomach in with force on the fourth step. Repeat for 3-4 minutes.

If you have too much pain to do this variation, squeeze without force and repeat for only one minute.

HIGH KNEE WALKING

Return to walking forward and backward with upright posture without the abdominal contractions (FIGURE 7). After you have attained

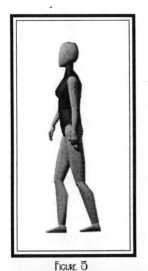

FIGURE 5

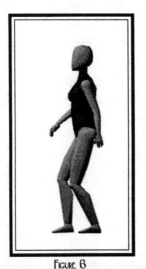

FIGURE 6

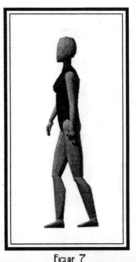

FIGURE 7

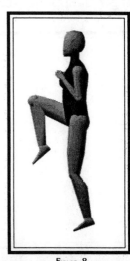

FIGURE 8

the alignment you desire, begin to lift the knee before each step. Gradually lift your knee as high as you can before stepping forward (FIGURE 8, P.33). Be sure your speed is slow enough to accomplish this move with good alignment and with no back strain. As the leg comes down from the kneelift, be sure to use the leg and buttocks muscles to do the job. Try not to tilt or feel any work in the back. If you can keep your spine upright, you'll know you're using the right muscles. This exercise will strengthen the hamstrings and gluteals.

LONG STRIDE WALKING

Return to walking forward and backwards with upright posture without the abdominal contractions. After you have attained the alignment you desire, begin to take longer strides. Cover more territory with fewer steps than you did before. As your strides get longer, think about keeping your ribs up and

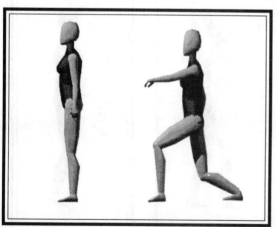

FIGURE 9

maintaining good alignment. The tendency will be to lean forward. Don't give in to it. Stay tall. Repeat for 2 minutes. This exercise is excellent for joint mobility and stretching the hip flexors.

POWER WALKING

Begin walking with shorter strides again but walk very slowly. As soon as you've slowed yourself down, begin to dip down to immerse your shoulders with each step. Be sure to move slowly enough to maintain correct alignment (FIGURE 9). The knees and hips bend while your torso stays upright. Continue power walking for 2-3 minutes. Power walking is an excellent way to strengthen the leg and buttocks muscles without creating a "load" on the back.

THE OBLIQUE ABDOMINAL MUSCLES

Do not do this exercise set if you've had a hip replacement unless you clear it with your physician or therapist.

Return to a slow "tall" walk moving forward and backwards. After you're sure you have the right alignment, begin a crossing walk (FIGURE 10, P.35). When moving forward cross each foot over the other when stepping forward. For example, step the right foot to the left side of the left foot before shifting your weight to it. When moving backwards, cross each foot behind the other.

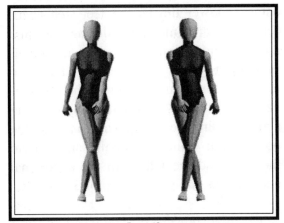

FIGURE 10

backing up, lift your leg slightly out to the side before crossing it behind the other foot. Keep the moves controlled and the body upright and strong. Continue this exercise for 3-4 minutes. This exercise further improves balance, and also works the abductors and adductors in the inner and outer thighs.

The last degree of difficulty for this exercise is to dip (immerse) the shoulders each time the feet come together to step down (FIGURE 12). Visualize good alignment, and work on

Mentally visualize yourself with good upright posture and continue this exercise for 3-4 minutes. This exercise works the midriff muscles and improves balance.

Continue the crossing walk but make it a little more difficult by lifting the leg slightly out to the side before bringing it down and crossing it over the other foot (FIGURE 11). When

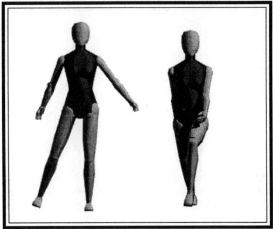

FIGURE 12

using power to push the shoulders out of the water on each leg lift. If possible, continue this exercise moving forward and backwards for 3 minutes. This exercise continues to

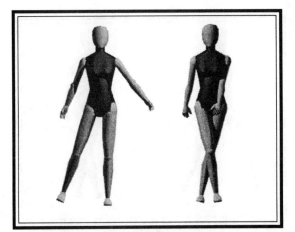

FIGURE 11

improve balance, adductors abductors, and adds strength and flexibility for the quadriceps, hamstrings (front and back of thighs), and gluteals

THIGHS AND ISOMETRIC ABDOMINAL WORK

Step sideways through the water, moving to the right at least 8 steps and then to the left. Keep your knees and toes pointed forward. Think about alignment. Continue for 2 minutes. This exercise works the adductors and abductors (inner and outer thighs).

Increase the intensity of this exercise by using a power dip as the feet step apart. Shoulders are immersed during the step apart, shoulders come out of the water during the step together (Figure 13). As feet step together, consciously contract the abdominal muscles. This can be done by thinking about pressing the stomach down toward the pool bottom. Continue stepping sideways to the right and the left, with the abdominal contractions and power dips for 3 minutes.

Do not do this exercise set if you've had a hip replacement unless you clear it with your physician or therapist.

Return to stepping sideways with no power dip. Cross the right foot over the left when moving to the left. Cross the left foot over the right when moving to the right (Figure 14). This is a sideways crossing step that develops balance, coordination, and muscular flexibility. Continue for 3 minutes.

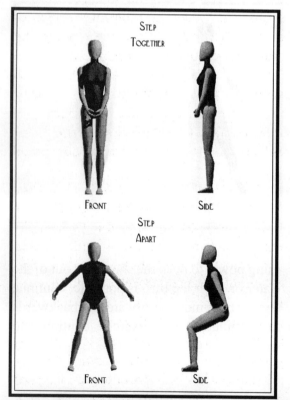

STEP
TOGETHER

FRONT   SIDE

STEP
APART

FRONT   SIDE

FIGURE 13

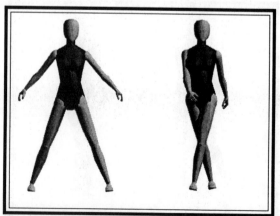

FIGURE 14

DEEP WATER WITH A VEST OR BELT

Put a flotation belt on. Move to the deep end of the pool.

NOTE: In the deep water it is easier to move if your body is leaning forward. DON'T LEAN FORWARD. Leaning forward will burn fewer calories and it will put excess strain on the low back. Keeping good postural alignment with the shoulders directly over the hips (from a side view) will make moving through the water more difficult (you'll burn more calories) and also cause the abdominal and back muscles to co-contract (you'll get safe strengthening for both).

HIGH-KNEE JOG

Jog easily forward and backwards through the water with high knees. Fluidly pull each knee up toward the chest, as high as possible, before pressing it straight down toward the pool bottom (FIGURE 15). Practice perfectly upright alignment. Do a breast-stroke with the arms while moving forward and a backstroke using both arms simultaneously while moving backwards. One powerful breaststroke or backstroke is used for every four jogs. Continue this exercise for 2 minutes.

After you feel you're accomplishing a good, upright high-knee jog, add the abdominal contraction on every fourth jog. Think about having a sponge in your stomach and squeezing it out on every fourth count. "Jog, jog, jog, squeeze." When the "squeeze" becomes comfortable, start to use the words "tall, tall, tall, squeeze" to return to good alignment. Repeat this moving forward and backwards for 3 minutes.

Note: You will not move very far forward or back with the jog, that's not the purpose.

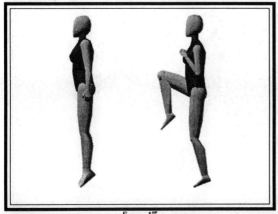

FIGURE 15

DOUBLE KNEE SCOOP

Continue moving forward with the high-knee jog, but move backwards with a double knee scoop. Begin with both knees up and out to their respective sides. As the arms move forward during the backstroke, powerfully squeeze both knees together (FIGURE 16, P.38). Knees will end up together in front of your chest. During the scoop, forcefully press the abdominals down toward the pool bottom. Remember to maintain good

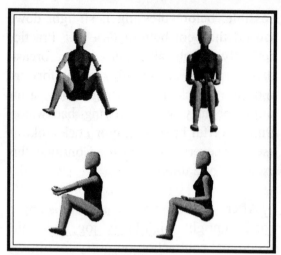

FIGURE 16

alignment and continue this (high-knee jog forward, double knee scoop backwards) for 3 minutes.

COOLDOWN

Relax your muscles by jogging easily forward and backwards in the deep water or walk easily in the shallow water. Continue to maintain good pelvic alignment but

eliminate the forceful or powerful moves. Jog or walk for two minutes.

FINAL STRETCHES

Finish the workout with calf, hamstring and hip flexor stretches in the shallow water.

Calf stretch. Face pool edge and hold pool edge. Take a step forward with one foot and lean slightly forward. Pull the toes of the back foot up. You should feel a nice stretch in the calf of the back leg. Hold the stretch about 10 to 15 seconds and then reverse to stretch the other leg.

Hamstring stretch. Pull your right knee up to your chest. Without leaning forward, straighten your right knee until you feel easy tension in the back of your right thigh. Hold for 10 to 15 seconds and reverse to stretch the other leg. You can do this stretch with your back to the pool wall or facing the pool wall with your foot balancing on the wall.

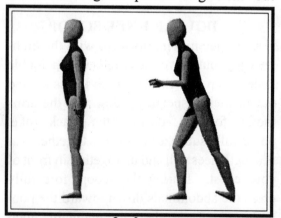

CALF STRETCH

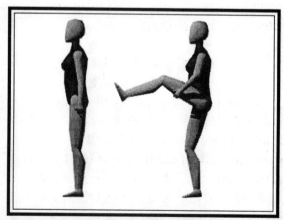

HAMSTRING STRETCH

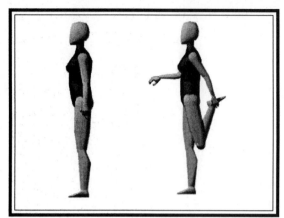

HIP FLEXOR STRETCH

Jog forward in the deep water by first pulling your knee up to your chest and then straightening it out in front of you before pulling it back (FIGURE 17). Alignment must be perfect and abdominals have to be contracted during the "straight leg pull back" to protect the low back. Go very slowly and with complete control. Do only for 1 minute.

Jog forward and backwards with straight legs. Rather than bending and straightening

Hip flexor stretch. Pull your right heel behind your right thigh. Allow your right knee to swing back just a bit until you feel a gentle stretch in the front of the hip. Go into a pelvic tilt and hold that position for 10 to 15 seconds and then reverse to stretch the left hip flexors.

Before exiting the pool, repeat the BACK STRETCHES AND ABDOMINAL TIGHTENING section (Figures 1 through 4) of the workout in either the deep or shallow end.

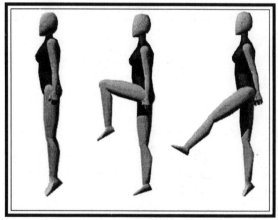

FIGURE 17

OPTIONAL EXERCISES
For the Brave of Back

As you are able to do these exercises without pain, you may want to add the following two additional moves. These exercises should not be added until you can accomplish all the preceding exercises without pain during the exercises or for two hours after the workout.

the knees, simply move the legs from the hips. Attempt to do this movement in place during the first workout session in which you try it. If no pain occurs afterwards, move it forward and backwards during the next workout. Do slowly only for one minute.

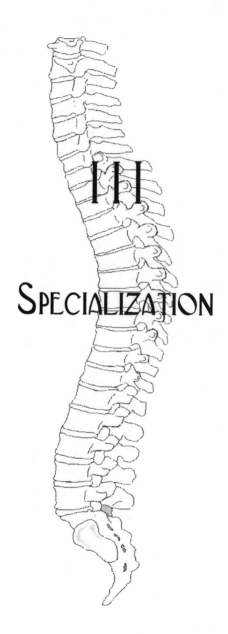

III

SPECIALIZATION

CHAPTER 8
ESPECIALLY FOR YOU
FASTBACK

If the back is fast (and fine) but a different body part is slow, BackHab can still work its magic. Here are some precautions and modifications for others who participate in the BackHab program.

BackHab for Clients With Arthritis

Arthritis means "joint inflammation" ("arth" = joint, "itis" = inflammation), and the term refers to more than 100 rheumatic diseases but the two major types are Osteo and Rheumatoid. Whether it's Osteo or Rheumatoid Arthritis the modifications of BackHab are the same. Arthritis is a chronic disease and it affects joints, muscles, and connective tissue. It is an inflammation of the joints characterized by pain, instability and a decreased range of motion.

The goals of using BackHab are to increase range-of motion, increase flexibility, increase muscular strength, increase value of life, and increase movement for activities of daily living.

Depth: Be sure affected joints are submerged. The hydrostatic pressure and buoyancy of the water will decrease the edema and joint compressive forces in the joint capsule.

Water Temperature: Clients with arthritis find temperatures of 86 to 92 degrees ideal. The warmer water assists in decreasing pain. Cooler water can be used with warmth-providing clothing (Wet Wrap vest or shorts, Kiefer neoprene gloves, etc.).

Equipment: Add equipment only with therapist/medical approval. Equipment that requires gripping should barely be used. Buoyant and resistive equipment create extra load or compressive forces on the joints.

Arthritis cont...

Barbells not only overload fingers (with gripping) but also overload wrists, elbows, shoulders and sometimes the spine. Ankle cuffs affect ankles, knees, hips and back.

Modifications:
- Add some fine motor skills (wrists, fingers, toes, ankles, neck) to the BackHab movements.

- The two-hour-pain rule applies (see Chapter Six for more information).

- Encourage easy full ROM (range of motion) of all joints.

- Keep control of all movements so the effort is in the muscles, not the joint.

BackHab for Clients With Asthma or COPD

The most common respiratory disorders are asthma, chronic bronchitis and emphysema, which are part of a group of diagnoses called chronic obstructive pulmonary disease (COPD). In clients with COPD, the lungs' ability to exchange air decreases, making breathing difficult.

Clients who suffer from lung diseases such as chronic bronchitis or emphysema usually have much more difficulty breathing during exercise than clients with asthma.

The majority of individuals with asthma also have a form of asthma known as exercise-induced asthma (EIA). Clients with EIA experience asthmatic symptoms following an exercise bout. Although encouraging clients with EIA to exercise may sound contradictory, researchers have found that exercise can improve their condition.

Depth: As the lungs experience the hydrostatic pressure of the water the muscles of inspiration (inhaling) have to work harder. This creates an excellent breathing exercise medium. However, clients may experience dyspnea (labored or distressed breathing) if the inspiratory muscles aren't conditioned enough to tolerate the extra pressure.

Use deeper water (armpit to shoulder) if possible but begin shallow (waist) and watch for distress as the depth is gradually increased. If distress occurs, move shallower and work in shallow water that day. Each day will be different regarding water depth tolerance because of varied allergens affecting the client.

Water Temperature: Any water temperature can work. Air quality, temperature and humidity are more important than water temperature. Warm, humid air is beneficial for these clients.

Modifications:

- Spend at least ten minutes warming up. Most clients who have distress during exercise have it within the first eight to ten minutes.

- Use nasal breathing. Inhaling into the nose warms and lubricates the air before it enters the lungs.

- Avoid food two hours prior to the BackHab program. Combining food (which may cause an allergic reaction) with the chlorine in the air could create problems.

- Drink water before, during and after the BackHab program. Staying hydrated is very important for these clients because mucus plugging can result from inadequate fluid intake.

- Make sure the bronchodilator (inhaler) is at pool edge. An inhaler locked in the locker room won't help a client who is experiencing an attack.

- Spend extra time between each BackHab exercise for rest. These clients do better with start-and-stop activities than with continual aerobic movement.

- Include some relaxation time with diaphragmatic breathing exercises at the end of the session. Diaphragmatic breathing against the hydrostatic pressure can not only strengthen the intercostals, but also create a parasympathetic response to allow these clients to relax.

BackHab for Clients With CVA

Cerebral Vascular Accidents (CVA) are also called Strokes, and are the most common neurological disorder in the United States. Results of an insult to the brain may be central nervous system changes (speech/language), judgment, perception alterations, and/or changes in voluntary motor (spasticity, flaccidity, loss of coordination, ataxic gait patterns and loss of muscular strength).

The goals of the BackHab program for CVA clients are balance improvement, postural muscle re-education and gait training (stride length, cadence, velocity, etc.).

Depth: Begin in shallow (waist to midriff) depth water. If balance is a major problem, it can be best achieved in shallower water. If, on the other hand, weight bearing is a major problem it can best be achieved in deeper water.

Assuming that balance is a problem, begin in shallow water to work on balancing skills. Move to deeper water to progress. Deeper water challenges balance more and will make balancing skills more difficult.

Equipment: You may need to use weights to anchor a flaccid limb, or buoyancy to assist in moving a spastic limb. Except for assistance with balance or postural skills equipment should not be added.

Water Temperature: Clients who are quite functional can manage in water temperatures 82 – 86. Clients who are slow moving will need warmer water temperatures of approximately 88 – 92 degrees.

Modifications:

- Spend most of the time on the BackHab walking exercises (not the strengthening or stretching). Research shows that exercising lower extremities (legs) greatly improves functional recovery.

- Move slowly to improve balance. If clients are quite functional and can do the BackHab exercises at a normal tempo, slow the movements down to challenge balance even more. Having to slow the movement down encourages accurate muscle reeducation and challenges balance.

- Watch for exhaustion. Even though these clients may be moving very slowly it can be exhausting for them to have only half of their muscles firing and have to drag "dead weight" along with
  them. Allow them to rest between the BackHab exercises.

- Use more "backing-up" movements. Reversing the skill often assists clients in being able to learn it. It also improves muscle imbalance, which is a major problem for these clients.

- Allow time for relaxation. Many of these clients experience muscle spasticity, which may improve with relaxation techniques (such as Ai Chi) or by simply allowing the limb to drag through the water resistance.

- Use water walking for prevention of second strokes. Research has shown that walking can significantly reduce the risk of stroke. After a client is able to move through the BackHab program use the water walking program (in this BackHab book) for health maintenance.

BackHab for Clients With Coronary Artery Disease

Coronary Artery Disease (CAD) and Coronary Heart Disease (CHD) are extremely common in the United States. Whether it's angioplasty, a by-pass, angina, athlersclerosis, ischemic heart disease, valve disease, cardiomyopathy or any other artery or heart disease the BackHab program can be used. The primary goals in the BackHab program are to reduce risk factors (smoking, hypertension, hypercholesterolemia, diabetes, and physical inactivity) and prevent myocardial ischemia and infarction. Regular aerobic exercise is an important therapy with the potential to impact all of these.

Depth: Begin with midriff depth (coincidentally also called heart depth) for clients with CAD/CHD. If they have no pulmonary or coronary distress at that depth it will be an ideal depth for them to work at. If they have distress you may have to move them shallower.

Water Temperature: Water temperatures from 82 – 90 degrees can work. Extreme temperatures are probably not good. Pools with temperatures of 78 (or on the other end at 98) could create too much of a shock to the system. Pools with cooler temperatures are excellent at allowing the client to exercise without creating additional heart stress from excess heat buildup. If clients work in warmer water (88 – 92 degrees) they should keep the BackHab program at a slow pace and watch for exhaustion.

Equipment: Most equipment increases blood pressure, which is not an indication for these clients. No equipment should be necessary for the BackHab program.

Modifications:
- Watch for breath holding. During the strengthening and stretching programs in the BackHab program these clients may hold their breath (this increases blood pressure). Cue these clients for a continuous regular breathing pattern.

- Watch for dizziness or chest pain. If clients experience dizziness or chest pain have them leave the water and rest. If the symptoms do not subside get medical help.

- Have fun with BackHab. Many of these clients are so worried that anything they do will be the last thing they do (it will kill them), that they forget to enjoy movement for movements sake. Find ways to play during the program.

- Work on posture. Many of these clients tend to internally rotate the shoulders and hang forward to protect the heart. Instead help them to press the shoulder blades down and open the rib cage so they have good air exchange in the lungs.

BackHab for Clients With Diabetes

The two most common metabolic disorders in the United States are obesity and diabetes. Many of the BackHab modifications for diabetes also pertain to obesity. Type I is called insulin-dependent diabetes and Type II is called adult-onset or non-insulin dependent diabetes. Because of inactivity many children now have Type II (adult-onset) diabetes.

The goal of the BackHab program is to lessen the fluctuation of blood glucose through exercise. The water is an ideal place for clients with diabetes because submersion increases circulation (and most clients with diabetes have poor circulation). These clients many also have vision problems and heart disease.

Depth: Clients with diabetes should practice the BackHab program at approximately midriff depth. They may need to move a little bit deeper to protect their feet from scraping the pool bottom if the pool bottom is rough.

Water Temperature: Water temperatures ranging from 82 – 92 degrees can work fine for clients with diabetes. Overheating in warm water should be avoided. If warm water is used the program should be slowed down and taken at an easy pace.

Modifications:

- Know the signs for hypoglycemia. These include:

√ anxiety and restlessness
√ irritability
√ nausea
√ extreme hunger
√ confusion
√ double vision
√ excessive sweating and heart palpitations

√ headache
√ loss of motor coordination
√ pale, moist skin
√ strong, rapid pulse

A client showing any of these symptoms should immediately stop exercising and consume a sweetened product.

• Have a simple carbohydrate at pool edge. Quickly available sugar includes five to six Life Savers, two tablespoons of honey, four sugar cubes or six to eight ounces of orange juice. Any of these will provide the 10 to 15 grams of sugar most frequently recommended.

• Clients should have a complex carb around the exercise program.

• Exercising too soon after taking insulin can result in serious problems, especially if a client takes too much insulin.

• Clients should self-test blood glucose levels. Clients should check blood glucose levels before activity and again four hours after exercise in order to monitor their response to the BackHab program.

• Clients should wear shoes. Foot ulcers are common in people with Type I diabetes and loss of lower extremity sensation is common with both kinds of diabetes. Clients may wear away more than a superficial layer of skin from their feet without being aware of it. Shoes will protect their feet.

BackHab for Clients With Fibromyalgia Syndrome (FMS)

Clients with fibromyalgia are constantly in a state of sympathetic (fight or flight) system arousal and their pain is traditionally in muscles not joints. For an FMS diagnosis clients must have pain and aching in many parts of the body lasting for at least 3 months and local tenderness in eleven of eighteen specified places on the body.

The goal of the BackHàb program is to provide exercise, slowly increased toward full cardiovascular conditioning, toning, and stretching in a low impact medium.

Depth: Clients with fibromyalgia may want to participate in the BackHab program at a bit deeper than midriff. Heart to shoulder depth may give them more relaxation and less pain.

Temperature: Water temperature from approximately 84 – 92 degrees can work well for a client with fibromyalgia.

Cold water is generally thought not to be good.
Extreme changes of temperature (moving from a cold water pool to a whirlpool and visa versa) would be contraindicated.

Clients should not work to exhaustion so if the water temperature is warm clients should take the BackHab program at a slow pace.

Modifications:
- Have clients work easily or "lightly". Clients with fibromyalgia tend to give 150%, which means they will use inappropriate and excessive muscle recruitment and often try to do too much. Keep them relaxed and playing easily with the BackHab program.

- Watch for fatigue. Tiredness is okay with an FMS client; exhaustion is not. Exhaustion can exacerbate their symptoms and create more pain. They are more likely to overdo because of their personalities.

- Add relaxation at the end of BackHab. Because of the sympathetic/parasympathetic balance these clients need to spend some time eliciting a parasympathetic response. That can be done with relaxation programs (such as Ai Chi) or simply with diaphragmatic breathing at the end of the BackHab session.

BackHab for Clients with Hip Replacements

Clients with hip replacements often come to the BackHab program limping or "vaulting" while walking. The goal of the BackHab program is to gradually re-educate the walking musculature so that the foot strike, stride, stride length, and rhythm are relearned correctly.

Depth: Clients with hip replacements should begin in deeper water (because of their weight bearing difficulties) and gradually, after several weeks, progress to shallower water.

Temperature: Clients with hip replacements manage well with water temperature 84 – 92 degrees. Water temperatures less than 84 degrees often create a muscle tension that will not allow the joint to function properly.

Equipment: Unless used for balance and posture, equipment should not be used for clients with hip replacements because of the excessive torque and shear forces in the joint.

Modifications:

- Shorten stride length. Clients who are "repatterning" need to begin with short strides to allow the   muscles to learn correct functioning. Eventually lengthen the stride, but only if the rest of the body maintains a controlled stature, balance, and the stride is still correct.

- Learn contraindications. Traditional contraindications include the elimination of crossing the midline, hip flexion beyond 90 degrees, and hip internal or external rotation. New surgeries involving incisions on different aspects of the hip may change

these contraindications. Many clients will be far enough post-op that they will have no contraindications.

- Work on balance and posture. Clients with hip replacements, much like clients with strokes, need to relearn balance skills and postural alignment. During the BackHab program focus on alignment issues. Review the Cerebral Vascular Accident modifications for balance ideas.

BackHab for Knee Injuries or Total Knee Replacements

Whether the situation involves cartilage injuries (such as meniscus tears), tendon injuries (such as patellofemoral pain syndrome), ligament injuries (such as ACL), osteoarthritis, or post surgery from TKR the modifications are similar. The goal of the BackHab program for clients with knee injuries or replacements is to work toward structural stability, flexibility, and strength while moving in functional patterns.

Depth: Water depth for clients with

knee injuries or replacements should be according to their tolerance. If there are serious weight-bearing issues the client should be deeper in the water to allow the buoyancy to assist. If clients don't have weight bearing issues midriff to armpit depth is ideal.

Temperature: Clients with knee injuries or replacements manage well with water temperature 84 – 92 degrees. Water temperatures less than 84 degrees often create a muscle tension that will not allow the joint to function properly.

Equipment: Unless used for balance and posture equipment should not be used for clients with knee injuries or replacements because of the excessive torque and shear forces in the joint.

Modifications:
- Move the leg as one unit. When moving laterally through the water the knee joint should be tightened so that the leg moves as one piece. If this is not done the water resistance can create torque and compressive forces in the joint.

- Slow the BackHab exercises down. While moving with high knees or hamstring curls it's im-

portant that the knee muscles have enough time to move the lower leg on a straight plane. If knee flexion is performed at regular speed the lower leg tends to zigzag through the movement.

- Focus on closed kinetic chain moves when possible. The dip (or squat) used in the BackHab program will be excellent for these clients. Having the foot connected to the pool bottom during the flexion and extension of the knee assists much like a joint-stabilization brace would.

- Work on balance techniques. Review balance techniques in the Cerebral Vascular Accident section of this chapter to assist these people in relearning balance.

BackHab for Clients with Muscular Sclerosis (MS)

MS is a neuromuscular disorder involving the gradual destruction of nerves (the nerve covering, known as the myelin sheath, is slowly destroyed) and muscles, which results in a progressive loss of movement. Helping to slow the progression of the disease and maintain lower extremity function is the goal of the BackHab program. People with MS should make exercise an integral part of their lives.

Depth: Clients with MS should work in as shallow water as possible. Because they may eventually lose sensation in the lower extremities it is important that they have neural feedback from those areas. Clients can start at midriff depth and, if balance, postural alignment and gait are fine, the clients can be moved shallower.

Temperature: Clients with MS have hypersensitivity to both internal and external temperature increases. Water temperature for these clients can range from 78 – 85 degrees. Warmer water can be used only if the client is moving very slowly and is quite passive.

Equipment: Unless used for balance and posture, equipment should not be used for clients with MS because of fatigue.

Modifications:
- Watch for fatigue. Clients with MS can fatigue easily either from increased body temperature, warm water or activity. The fatigue will reduce their mobility.

- Watch for overheating. Clients with MS are hypersensitive to temperature increases. Movement or exercise create energy which has a by-product of heat. Keep the BackHab program and at an even pace. Heat can create a temporary loss of function in these clients.

- Work on gait training and balance. The loss of myelin results in less controlled and more uncoordinated movement. Maintaining balance while moving with correct patterns will assist these clients in maintaining function.

- Move slowly. Slow movement in the water can assist in maintaining the neural pathways that lead to coordinated movement patterns.

BackHab for Obese Clients

Obesity is the number one metabolic disease in the United States. Traditional overweight clients can participate in the BackHab program safely without modifications. Morbidly obese clients will need modifications.

Depth: Clients should begin in midriff to armpit depth to eliminate as much impact as possible. However, be aware that these clients might easily lose control of their movements and may have to be moved shallower to increase control.

Temperature: Morbidly obese clients are best in temperatures from 78 - 84 degrees. It is generally thought they should not participate in a BackHab program in water temperatures over 86. Obese clients have difficulties with heat dissipation and the combination of heat buildup from movement within the body and the heat of the water can create an overheating situation.

Modifications:
- Watch for hypernea, dyspnea and apnea. Obese clients will sometimes present with fast breathing (hypernea) or distressed breathing (dyspnea). If that occurs clients should rest between each of the BackHab exercises.

- Other clients may present with apnea during some of the toning, strengthening or stretching exercises. Apnea is breath holding and should be discouraged.

- Teach clients "recovery to stand". Because of the buoyancy these clients have they are more likely to tip,

lose their footing and not be able to regain an upright posture. Have them practice returning to upright position from supine and prone flotation.

- Watch for overheating. Obese clients tend to use more energy in movement patterns which creates more heat. Their heat dissipation abilities are compromised because of the layers of insulation beneath their skin. Begin very gradually with the BackHab program and keep all movements at a low intensity.

BackHab for Osteoporosis

Osteoporosis is a metabolic bone disease that gradually reduces bone mass and leads to pain, especially in the back, hips and neck. The goal of the BackHab program is to allow these clients a safe and supportive exercise medium while assisting in the maintenance of bone density. Modifications for osteopenia are the same.

Depth: These clients may need the extra support of deeper (armpit) water but will benefit also from midriff depth.

Temperature: Water temperatures from 80 – 84 degrees work well with clients with osteoporosis. If they are frail and slow moving, warmer water temperatures will be necessary.

Equipment: If clients are functional enough to be able to move easily with the BackHab program there's a possibility that resistant equipment can assist in their goals. Experiment first with webbed gloves while participating in the BackHab program. Progress from there as tolerated.

Modifications:
- Avoid jerky movements. Clients with osteoporosis need to use forceful movements in the water but not jerky movements. Adding a "stop and start" to each of the BackHab movements will assist these clients. The "stop and start" technique will make the ligaments in the joint create a tug on the periosteum at the end of the bone, which initiates the resorption and remodeling process.

- Require shoes. Clients with osteoporotic bones will often shatter bones if they fall. The deck and locker room contain hard, slippery surfaces. Requiring shoes from the locker room into the pool and back will protect these clients.

- Work on postural alignment. Clients with osteoporosis will have less pain if they can get the bones stacked properly. Using and strengthening muscles in proper alignment will assist them in maintaining postural alignment through their activities of daily living.

BackHab for Clients With Shoulder Injuries and Pain

It is thought that 70% of the population in the United States has asymptomatic shoulder problems. Many of these problems come because the subacromial space becomes diminished because of internal shoulder rotation in everyday posture. The goal of the BackHab program is to move without pain, and with proper structural alignment to open the subacromial.

Depth: Clients who have shoulder problems should have the shoulders submerged. The hydrostatic pressure and buoyancy will decrease the edema and joint compressive forces in the joint capsule. Moving through the BackHab program with shoulders submerged will slow the client down but will be very beneficial.

Temperature: Water temperatures ranging
from 84 – 92 degrees work well with clients
with shoulder problems. Warmer water will
lessen the tension in the muscles and thereby
lessen the pain.

Equipment: No equipment should be used
for clients with shoulder injuries and pain.

Modifications:
- Let the arms drag. When moving forward in the BackHab program, allowing the arms to drag behind will open
  the shoulder joint capsule and the
  subacromial space.

- Depress the scapulae. Pressing the
  shoulder blades down lightly will assist in getting the shoulders and upper trunk into better alignment.

- Use hands behind the back. Walking forward, backwards or sideways
  with hands behind the back will
  strengthen the trunk and keep the
  scapula in proper positioning.

- Use external shoulder rotation. While
  moving through the BackHab program vary the arms so that external
  shoulder rotation occurs.

CHAPTER 8
ANCHORS AWEIGH
SOLID TO THE CORE

Alignment is the most important aspect of BackHab. Alignment is the focus and is required before any movement is implemented. This chapter will take postural structural alignment into more depth.

BackHab treats the body as a highly integrated structure instead of a series of independent parts. Rather than exercising by moving one limb, BackHab incorporates that limb movement into full body mobility. Adding the core stability concept (anchoring) to the BackHab program can double the benefits to clients.

As we age and go through the different movements in our lives, these movements create postural and structural changes. Some of our muscles get shorter and broader in diameter, some of them lose tension and become longer and stretched out, some become tight and taunt, and others retain elasticity. The changes in these muscles will create changes in biomechanical movement and therefore result in other muscles compensating and changing. These changes eventually affect joint mechanics which can lead to a decrease in functional movement. The core stability concept can help us take our clients back to more functional movement.

Concepts of Core Stability

The core, often called the trunk, is the body's center of power. All movement should be initiated from the core. For this to happen muscles must work to stabilize the spine and pelvis, and reestablish a proper sequence of muscle firing patterns. In core stability the stabilizers should fire before the prime movers.

Core stability allows us to stabilize proximally to allow for safe and efficient distal movement. This will decrease stress to ligaments, intervertebral discs and joint structures. Proper recruitment patterns need to occur before the movement begins.

What does this all mean? It means that before the legs move, the abdominal and gluteal muscles need to contract to stabilize; and the scapula and upper trunk muscles stabilize before the arms move. This is also called moving from the "inside out". When we're born we initiate all movement from the trunk. Eventually our bodies adapt and learn to move in the easiest way. That's when we begin moving our arms and legs without first anchoring the trunk. You will see this in clients when they move the extremities and cause the body to "wag".

How To Implement Core Stability

Here's a simple way to incorporate core stability into the BackHab program. Try anchoring while walking forward and backwards. Start walking with a normal alignment and stride. Pull your stomach in. Now pull it in a little more. Keep walking and now think about pulling your stomach up toward your ribs. Keep holding your stomach in and consciously breathe into and out of the rib cage.

Pull your stomach in a little more and up a little higher. Now inhale into the rib cage while continuing to pull your stomach in and up, but exhale from the diaphragm. Isn't it amazing that you can contract the transversus even more? Continue walking with abdominals in and up while inhaling into the rib cage (while pulling your stomach in and up) and exhaling from the diaphragm. The transverse abdominals are now engaged.

Keep them contracted. Don't relax yet. Now you have one part of core stability – *the deep tissue abdominals*. Go ahead and contract your abdominals more but remember to keep your alignment upright. The rib cage is lifted and chin is back as you continue to walk. Pull your stomach in a little tighter. Hold it in.

Relax. Aaaah. Doesn't that feel good?

Now think about pressing the scapula down toward your back hip pockets while you're walking. Press them down a little harder. You're not squeezing them together; you're pushing the scapula as low as they'll go. Start with the lateral aspect of your thumbs at your waist just behind the side-view midline. Slide your thumbs down your hips to your thighs. When your thumbs won't go any further the scapula are in proper alignment.

You may feel tightness in the upper trapezius and pectorals (that's okay, they probably need the stretching) and your neck will look longer as your shoulders slope down. Continue walking with the scapula depressed.

Now you have another part of core stability – *scapular alignment*. Press them down harder while you continue walking with strong upright alignment. Chin is back and abdominals are lifted. Keep going.

Relax. Aaaah. I love "relax".

Now contract the gluteals. Once they're contracted, squeeze them together as tightly as you can. Continue walking but allow the contraction to control your stride length. (The contraction will impede hip flexion.) Contract the gluteals more and squeeze them together more tightly.

Practice walking with the gluteals contracted. Remind yourself every ten seconds to contract harder. The hip and knee joints should still be able to flex and extend but the range of motion of the hip joint will be limited. That's okay.

This is another part of core stability – *gluteal contraction.* Continue walking and contract tighter. Remember that the rib cage is lifted and chin back. Feel strong, long and lean and continue walking.

Relax. Aaaah. Did I mention I love "relax"?

Now you have the concepts integrated into a basic stride. Try core stability with some of the BackHab strides and with edge of the pool muscular endurance work.

Strengthen from the inside out for better health, better alignment, better core conditioning and better caloric consumption.

Eventually, when clients are better able to coordinate the firing of their muscles, you can *combine the three core aspects.* Are you ready for more?

Begin walking again and press the scapulae down. Push them down lower until it feels like they can't go any further. Chin is back (not up) and rib cage should be lifted. Depress the scapulae a little more. Keep them down and pull your stomach in.

Think about a sponge full of water in your stomach. Now squeeze all the water out of the sponge and hold the sponge in squeezed position. Keep your shoulder blades down. Pull the sponge (that still has no water in it) up toward your rib cage and hold that position. Chin is still back and shoulder blades are depressed harder. Pull your stomach in and up a little more. Now squeeze your gluteals together. Squeeze harder. You can squeeze even harder. That's good, now hold them tight and don't let them relax. The stomach is still pulled in and up … go ahead and pull it in a little more.

Check to be sure the scapulae are down as low as they'll go and tighten the gluteals a lot more. Try to contract the buttocks so much that they can't get any tighter … and hold them there. Keep walking with your chin back, stomach in a little more, scapulae pressed down (don't forget them) and get your gluteals back to the tightness they were before. That's core stability. Hold a little more and …

Relax. Aaaah!

This is the kind of script you can use with clients. Constantly remind them of each aspect because as soon as they start to concentrate on one body part, the other part relaxes. The relaxation occurs because of lack of concentration, lack of training and natural muscular fatigue. We aren't used to having our deep tissue, core muscles working so hard.

The hope is that anchoring will eventually become natural, comfortable (!), and automatic.

At a certain point some of the muscles will develop new memory and deep tissue muscles will fire before extremity movement (without conscious thought) to protect the body and keep it looking long, lean, lithe and strong.

Some clients will walk out of a half-hour session are already looking taller and stronger.

Don't be afraid to give clients "homework".

Cliets can practice core concepts at home, at work, in the car, etc. but give them some hints to remind them of their homework. Use reminder cues like, "every time you get in the car, each time you look at your watch today, when you're standing in line, when you're in a meeting, every time you feel bored," to help them remember when to practice their homework.

The Benefits of Core Stability

Alignment, balance and kinesthetic awareness are all used and challenged when core stability concepts are used. Integration and coordination of movement and stability occurs (eventually) in the entire body.

- *Alignment* - When using the BackHab program with the core stability concepts, alignment is involved even more than with the traditional program. It becomes easier for clients to establish neutral spine. That decreases stress to the joints, muscles, tissue and vertebrae. Clients begin to work from the "inside out" with emphasis on the initiation of core muscles prior to movement of the extremities. The BackHab exercise movements become proximal to distal.

  Usually strong muscles become stronger and weak become weaker. The core stability concept prevents that from occurring.

- *Balance* - Not only does our body's dynamic alignment begin to improve when using the core stability concepts but balance improves too. Balance skills, both static and dynamic are equally important. Without balance we cannot sit, stand, walk or participate in activities of daily living.

Balance is a learned skill. Balance learned in the water (an unstable environment) translates well to land. When the trunk becomes stronger it can support the body in varied positions and movements.

- *Kinesthetic Awareness* – By "scheduling" movements to occur from the inside out, clients are able to improve their awareness of where their bodies are in space. They increase their proprioceptive awareness from the peripheral to the central nervous system. They have increased input into the central nervous system, which provides the musculoskeletal system with increased information on how to coordinate and control movements.

Since proprioception is the sum of input from all sensory receptors, increasing information to the central nervous system leads to greater awareness of the position of the body and limbs. This increases proprioceptive or kinesthetic awareness.

Proprioceptive trace is an after-effect of the immediate proprioceptive experience, which can be built on in successive BackHab classes.

Teaching Techniques

Hints
Here are some hints to help you use the concept with your clients.

- Do only a few repetitions using perfect technique. Poor technique can cause injury.
- Minimize mental and physical overload. Try only two or three exercises using the core stability concept at each session.
- Try only one aspect (stomach, scapula or gluteal squeeze) of the stabilization at a time. Remember that the primary mover is not the focus. Stabilizers and synergists engage first and should be felt internally anchoring the body.
- Encourage axial elongation during movement patterns.
- Provide detailed verbal and tactile cues to encourage awareness of precise skeletal alignment throughout movement.

Cues That Might Help You
Here are some cues to help you use the core stability concept with your clients.

To facilitate scapula depression
- Slide shoulder blades down toward your hip pockets
- Slide thumbs down your hips and back portion of outer thighs
- Press your shoulders down toward your waist

To facilitate contraction of abdominals with emphasis on activation of transversus
- Draw pelvic floor up toward the top of head
- Draw navel in and up toward the back of the waist
- Squeeze the water out of the sponge
- Hollow out your stomach

To facilitate gluteal contraction
- Accentuate your gluteal "smile" lines
- Squeeze your gluteals together
- Hold tightly to a hundred dollar bill between your buttocks

Common Errors
Situations you'll need to watch clients for include

- apnea (breath holding)
- shoulder elevation (keep shoulders relaxed)
- poor technique (decrease repetitions or find new verbal or tactile cues)
- chin forward (maintain neutral spine)
- moving too quickly

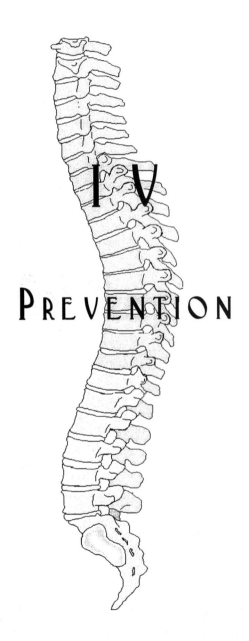

IV

PREVENTION

CHAPTER 10
STRAIGHT UP
AN OUNCE OF PREVENTION

O nce we are pain free it's difficult to be motivated to keep up with a preventative exercise program. To that Dr. Imrie (Goodbye Backache) says, "exercises are boring but, then, so is lying in bed with a backache." What can you do?

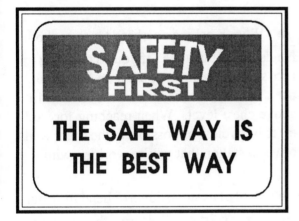

Relearn Activities of Daily Living

It is important to think of back safety during your daily situations. Many times our back problems stem from poor habits. Here are some helpful hints. Read through them today and then re-read one each day to keep some type of back health in the forefront of your mind.

Stay away from, or take a class to learn to work with, the negative stressors in your life.

Learn to use the "pelvic tilt" during all activities. To practice learning the pelvic tilt, stand with your back to the wall with your heels a few inches from the wall. Pull in your stomach muscles slightly, soften your knees (make sure they aren't locked), press your low back, shoulders and head against the wall and look straight ahead. This is the pelvic tilt position. Think about how this feels (besides uncomfortable!) and try to go into this position several times a day. This will allow the back to stretch and relax even while you're working.

Learn to stand so that your skeleton and muscles are efficiently doing the job. Stand tall, chin in, (avoid slouching or leaning), ribs up, shoulders centered, head over spine, back slightly flattened and knees slightly bent or "soft". If you must stand for a long period of time, try to put one foot on a low shelf and switch feet every now and then. Stand close to any work you must do and keep your arms at waist height.

Learn to sit with your knees even with or higher than your hips, with a slight low back curve, with your chin in, ribs up, shoulders centered, and without slouching. Try to use a chair that has a firm seat and supports the low back. Sit close to your work so you don't need to lean forward. It's okay to cross your legs as long as they don't get numb. Crossing your legs puts you in a natural pelvic tilt.

Drive using many of the same ideas of sitting. Move the seat back before getting out or in and then slide it close to the wheel to drive. Use your hands low on the wheel to rest the arms and upper back. If you're on a long trip, use cruise control to let you change leg positions. Get out and walk for awhile every hour.

Sleep or lie down in a position that allows you to maintain the natural curves in the spine. A fairly firm mattress usually works best. A mattress that is too firm doesn't allow heavier or larger parts of the body in sink into it. This can cause unnatural curvature. Lie on your back or sides. Try not to lie on your stomach.

Back strain often occurs from getting into or out of bed. If this causes problems for you, move the height of your bed up to sitting height.

While walking up and down stairs be sure to use the handrail and maintain correct posture. Leaning forward while going upstairs is not recommended. Also, don't pull yourself up by the handrail.

When reaching overhead try to use both hands rather than one. If you're reaching to take something down or put it up, you should use a stable stool so you don't have to lift above chest level. When reaching forward try to be as close as possible to the shelf, wall or work station that you're working with.

Most of us stoop down or bend from our hips or waist. Relearn the bending technique. Try to keep your back straight (shoulders over your hips) and use your knees to get you down and up instead. Bend with one knee in front of, or lower than the other. You may find that kneeling on one knee is necessary. You may also want to use your arms to get back up.

📌 Using long handled tools such as rakes, shovels, vacuum cleaners, mops, brooms, lawn mowers, paint rollers, etc. can be very stressful to the back. A simple rule of thumb is to move your feet with the tool rather than stretching your arms.

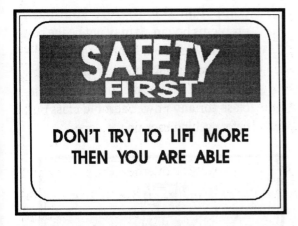

DON'T TRY TO LIFT MORE
THEN YOU ARE ABLE

📌 Lift only those items that you are strong enough to move. Improper lifting puts a tremendous compressive force on the discs of the low back. The discs will eventually weaken after repeated abuse and you will experience back pain. The National Safety Council recommends less than 30 pounds for women, and less than half the body weight for men. Keep the load close to the body. Be sure to use the proper bending techniques when lifting.

📌 When carrying, be sure that the item is close to your body and that your load is balanced. Use assistance whenever possible. If you must carry to one side such as a briefcase or a shoulder bag, move the load to the other side for an equal amount of time. Backpacks are ideal. Maintain proper posture while carrying.

📌 When turning or twisting try to move the feet and the entire body in that direction. Quick or repeated turning or twisting from the knees, waist or shoulders could cause problems. If you do need to turn or twist be sure to maintain good alignment.

📌 Sports. Stay active but only with "safe" sports. Some examples are walking, jogging, hiking and swimming. Here are some helpful hints:

Walking, cross country skiing and hiking are usually okay. Begin easily at first. Stay away from steep inclines and declines and watch yourself for perfect alignment.

Jogging can be okay if you gradually work up to a jog from a walk AND you can do it in excellent postural alignment. Again, try to stay away from steep inclines and declines.

Swimming can be okay but the back stroke and the sidestroke are the best. Go slowly for longer periods rather than several sets of speed followed by rest. The overhand crawl or breaststroke can be tried for short periods of time to test your body's ability to tolerate it. The butterfly shouldn't be used.

Sports like baseball, softball, basketball, ping-pong, horseback riding, ice skating and back packing are moderately okay. Participate cautiously and in moderation. Begin with only 10 to 15 minutes and, if you are pain-free for the next 24 hours, gradually increase the time you participate.

If you want to golf you should use a push cart for your clubs and ALWAYS push it in front of you, not pull it behind. Relax during the game. If you can't relax, you probably shouldn't participate. Don't lean backwards at the completion of your stroke. Remember alignment.

Bowling might be okay. Test it for a short period of time at first. Work on easily releasing the ball. Jerking backwards during the release can be stressful on the back.

Tennis might be okay. Watch your alignment and begin slowly with someone who will play easily, not competitively, with you. Be careful of arching your back during the overhead shots and the serve.

Skiing can be okay if you were a competent skier before your back problems began. It may not be the best thing if you're a beginner. Take it cautiously and stay away from bumpy surfaces. Take a ski conditioning class (or any power aerobic class) before getting back on the slopes.

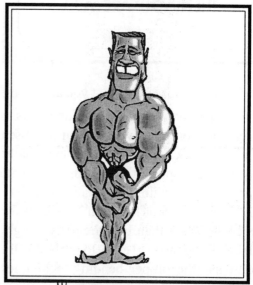

WEIGHTLIFTING SHOULD NOT CAUSE PAIN.

Weight lifting can be okay if the instructor knows and understands about your back problems. Begin with very light weights and do nothing that causes your back to arch or feel any strain. Keep your weights close to your body and move with control.

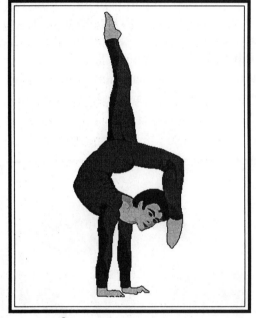

GYMNASTICS CAN CAUSE BACK DISTRESS.

The following sports should probably not be attempted. They usually involve a lot of twisting, turning, sudden impact, bouncing, contact or direct stress on the back.

Football
Touch football

Soccer
Gymnastics
Volleyball
Handball
Racquetball
Trampoline
Bungee jumping
Tobogganing
Sledding
Snowmobiling
Ice or field hockey

Guidelines For Good Nutrition

In 1979 the United States Food and Drug Administration developed classifications of foods into four broad groupsbased on certain key nutrients. The groups include: fruits and vegetables, grain products, milk and milk products, meats and meat substitutes. While recommendations for number of servings per day from each group vary based on age and growth development, a recommended average diet includes the following: fruits and vegetables 4 servings daily, grain products (breads and cereals) 4 servings daily, milk and milk products 2 servings daily, meats and meat substitutes 2 servings daily.

The recommended servings from the basic four food groups furnish approximately 1200-1500 calories per day and adequate amounts of essential nutrients if a variety of foods are selected.

In 1977 the Senate Agricultural Subcommittee on Nutrition set dietary guidelines to improve the health and quality of life of the American people.

The recommendations include:

1. Avoid becoming overweight by consuming only as much energy (calories) as you can expend. If you are overweight, decrease your energy intake and increase your energy expenditure.

2. Eat enough complex carbohydrates and "naturally occurring" sugars to account for about 40% of your energy intake. Do this by eating fresh fruits, vegetables, whole grains and products made with stone ground flour. Restrict the intake of the fine sugars and fruits that contain sucrose, corn sugar and corn syrup.

3. Limit your overall fat consumption to approximately 30% of your energy intake. Restrict consumption of saturated fats by choosing meats, poultry, fish and dairy products that are low in saturated fat. Restrict consumption of saturated fats to about 10% of the total energy intake with polyunsaturated fats accounting for 20%.

4. Maintain your cholesterol consumption at about 300 mg. per day by controlling the amount of milk products, eggs and butter fat consumed.

5. Limit your intake of sodium to less than five grams per day by controlling your consumption of salt and processed foods.

6. Reduce your consumption of artificial colorings, artificial flavorings, thickeners, preservatives and other food additives.

In 1979 the Department of Agriculture and the Department of Health and Human Services published a document titled "Nutrition and Your Health, Dietary Guidelines for Americans" which is the source for the following recommendations:

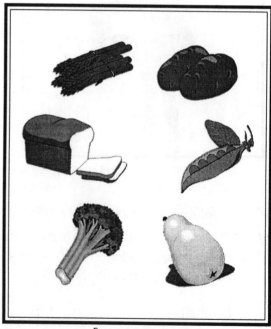

EAT A VARIETY OF FOODS

1. Eat a variety of foods daily including selections of fruits; vegetables; whole grain and enriched breads, cereals, grain products; milk, cheese, and yogurt; meats, poultry, fish and eggs; and legumes (dry peas and beans).

2. Maintain acceptable body weight by losing excess body weight and improving eating habits. To lose weight: increase physical activity, eat less fat and fatty foods, eat less sugar and sweets, and avoid too much alcohol. To improve eating habits: eat slowly, prepare smaller portions, and avoid "seconds."

3. Avoid too much fat, and saturated fat, and cholesterol. Choose lean meat, fish, poultry, dry beans and peas as your protein sources. Moderate your use of eggs and organ meats (liver). Limit your intake of butter, cream, hydrogenated margarines, shortenings and coconut oil, and foods made from such products. Trim excess fat off meats. Broil, bake, or boil rather than fry. Read labels carefully to determine both amount and types of fat contained in foods.

4. Eat foods with adequate starch and fiber: substitute starches for fats and sugars, and select foods that are good sources of fiber and starch, such as whole-grain breads and cereals, fruits and vegetables, beans, peas, and nuts.

5. Avoid too much sugar. Use less of all sugars, including white sugar, brown sugar, raw sugar, honey and syrups. Eat less food containing these sugars, such as candy, soft drinks, ice cream, cakes and cookies. Select fresh fruits or fruits canned without sugar or light syrup rather than heavy syrup. Read food labels for clues on sugar content -if the names sucrose, glucose, maltose, dextrose, lactose, fructose, or syrups appear first, then there is a large amount of sugar. And remember, how often you eat sugar is as important as how much sugar you eat.

6. Avoid too much sodium. Learn to enjoy the unsalted flavors of foods. Cook with only small amounts of added salt. Add little or no salt to foods at the table. Limit your intake of salty foods, such as potato chips, pretzels, salted nuts and popcorn, condiments (soy sauce, steak sauce, garlic salt), cheese, pickled foods, and cured meats. Read food labels to carefully determine amounts of sodium in processed foods and snack items.

7. If you drink alcohol, do so in moderation. Refrain from sustained or heavy drinking (more than two drinks per day).

Weight Control

A change in dietary habits or physical activity will aid in weight control and weight loss. A combination of diet and exercise will result in the ultimate weight loss program.

By eating 100 fewer calories a day and by walking for 30 minutes five times a week, a person could lose 22 pounds per year. People who incorporate regular aerobic exercise in a weight loss program lose more weight than those who do not.

Combining diet and exercise protects against the loss of lean tissue, eliminates the constant hunger and psychological stress of food deprivation and allows for flexibility in a weight loss regimen.

CHAPTER 11

WE'RE ALL WET

AQUATIC EXERCISE

Researchers at the University of Florida College of Medicine found that they produced excellent back pain relief results simply by strengthening the low back muscles. If low back workouts are effective in treating low back problems, they should be equally effective for preventing low back problems. "Low back distress is, to a surprising degree, preventable." (Westcott) So we know we should exercise. What can we do?

Ralph LaForge says that an ounce of prevention (exercise) can help avoid an aching back. He recommends a backache prevention program as including three components: aerobic exercise, flexibility exercises, and strengthening exercises. The workout in Chapter Ten "Beyond BackHab" will provide all three components.

Technical Stuff
Guidelines have been set by the American College of Sports Medicine for aerobic exercise programs. Be sure to follow them.

Begin with a gradual warm up, then go into the aerobic portion (explained below), then a cooldown and some stretching.

The aerobic portion of the workout is considered the "calorie burning portion". The goal of this section is to improve the cardiorespiratory system. The American College of Sports Medicine has made recommendations for developing and maintaining fitness in the healthy adult. These guidelines regarding the duration (length of each workout), intensity (how challenging the workout is for the cardiorespiratory system), frequency (how many times a week the workout should be repeated) and mode (the type of exercise necessary) of an aerobic exercise (cardiorespiratory) workout. If the workout does not meet the guidelines for each of these four aspects, it is not considered to be a cardiorespiratory or aerobic workout.

Mode

The ACSM (American College of Sports Medicine) guidelines state that the mode must be a large muscle activity, maintained continuously and rhythmical in nature. This means that the legs must be moving continuously for conditioning to occur. According to these guidelines a workout using only upper body movements would not qualify as aerobic.

Duration

The ACSM guidelines say that each workout should have an continuous aerobic portion lasting between 20 and 60 minutes. Twenty to thirty minutes is the average.

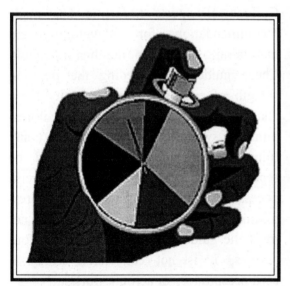

AVERAGE AEROBIC WORKOUT IS 20 TO 30 MINUTES LONG.

Intensity

The ACSM guideline states that the exercise intensity of the aerobic portion should be in a range of 50% to 85% of maximum heart rate reserve or Somewhat Hard to Hard on Borg's Rate of Perceived Exertion Chart. Find your ideal intensity on either the Heart Rate Chart or the Perceived Exertion Chart.

Borg's Rate of Perceived Exertion (RPE) Chart	
6	
7	Very, very light
8	
9	Very light
10	
11	Fairly light
12	
13	Somewhat hard
14	
15	Hard
16	
17	Very hard
18	
19	Very, very hard
20	

Source: Borg, G. A. V. (1982). Psychophysical Bases of Physical Exertion. *Medicine and Science in Sport and Exercise*, 14, 344-387. Used with permission.

Aquatic Exercise Association Aquatics Heartrate Chart

Age	Minimum Working Heartrate	Maximum Working Heartrate
20-29	124	179
30-39	119	161
40-49	114	152
50-59	108	143
60-69	103	134
70+	98	125

Checking Heartrates

Take Pulses after vigorous exercise to determine how hard the heart has worked.

1. As soon as exercise ceases, place the tips of the index and middle fingers lightly over one of the blood vessels on the neck (carotid arteries) located to the left or right of the Adam's apple.
2. Count the pulsations for six seconds, add a zero to the number, and refer to the chart.
3. If the pulse is below the target zone, exercise a little harder next time. If it is above the target zone, exercise should be lightened. If it falls within the target zone, exercise is taking place at the correct intensity.

Source: AEA, Nokomis, Florida

Frequency

The ACSM guidelines state that the workout should occur three to five times a week in order for results to occur.

WORK OUT 3 TO 5 TIMES A WEEK.

What About Osteoporosis

Regular vigorous will help osteoporosis. As you recall, osteoporosis was one of the causes of back problems. Bone mineral loss in the back bones generally begins in the mid-30's and is usually not reversible. It can, however, be retarded. Regular exercise and a diet rich in calcium can retard bone mineral loss. Smoking, crash diets, and extreme thinness will increase the speed of bone mineral loss.

The process of bone mineral loss is called osteoporosis which means porous bones. Osteoporosis affects women more often than men. White, small-boned, post-menopausal women (or women who stop menstruating due to over-training) are at the highest risk.

Originally it was thought the exercise had to be weight bearing (walking, running, aerobic dance) to have a beneficial affect on bone density. Research then found that a tennis player's dominant arm has more bone density than the other arm. Now it is known that stress on the tendons, ligaments and the periosteum (the place in the bone where new bone cells are made) is what triggers the increase in bone density.

Pushing and pulling limbs through the resistance of the water can assist in building or maintaining bone density. The beneficial stress can occur from the muscles contracting forcefully and pulling on the bone. The

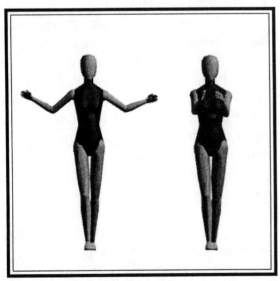

WATER RESISTANCE

stress can also occur from the impact of running on land or in the water, or the impact of hitting a ball with a racquet or pulling equipment through the water.

A bone subjected to continuous and excessive loads will grow thicker and stronger (remodel) as long as there is adequate nutrition, particularly calcium and phosphorus, and adequate periods of rest.

Bones that are not used become gradually weakened. Bones that are subjected to responsible exercise become stronger and denser. Exercise, then, can retard osteoporosis and stave off back problems caused by it.

Contraindicated Exercises

If you decide to stay in shape with an exercise program you'll want to understand contraindicated exercises. "Contraindicated" means that the exercise could be harmful to your physical well-being.

There are general high risk areas in the average body. Be aware of these specific areas to protect. High risk areas include the knees, the shoulders, the neck, and the low back.

Knees

The knees can be protected by remembering that moves that are safe for the knee joint will not straighten it too far, twist it, move it too quickly or bend it too far.

Use "soft" knees (knees which are in a slightly flexed position) throughout the workout to protect from straightening them too much.

A rule of thumb to protect the knee joint from twisting is to keep the knee and toes of the same foot pointed in the same direction at all times. If the knee is pointed out, the toes are also pointed out. If the knee is pointed forward, the toes are also pointed forward.

Movements should be slow and controlled when the knee joint is involved.

Shoulders

Seventy percent of our population has degenerative shoulder problems. Shoulder problems can occur when you spend a long time hanging from your arms on kickboards, buoyant jugs or from the edge of the pool. Exercises of this type should be done for only a short period of time before changing to another exercise which allows your shoulders to move back into their normal position.

Excessive use of the arms overhead, vigorous use of the arms overhead and use of weights with the arms overhead can all increase the likelihood of shoulder (and back) injuries. Using buoyant jugs that are partially filled with water as weights overhead is an extremely unstable move for the shoulders and should not be done.

Moving arms from below the surface of the water to above needs to be slow, controlled and should occur near the body rather than away from it.

Neck

The cervical vertebrae and discs can be aggravated during exercise. Hyperextension of the neck (looking straight up) should be eliminated. Fast, jerky moves in the neck can also damage the vertebrae and discs. Keep all the moves controlled and simple.

Lower Back

Hyperextension (arching) should be eliminated from your program. Flutter kicks, high kicks, kicking with both legs at once, and moving too quickly through the water can cause hyperextension of the low back. These moves should be eliminated. If you participate in a back strengthening program, you may do some back arching for back strengthening and abdominal stretching. If so, the moves should be extremely slow and controlled.

All the movements that involve the low back in any way should be slow and controlled with no jerky, quick movements.

For Land Based Exercises Eliminate:

>>: Situps either with the legs straight or bent. The curl-up, also called the trunk curl, is safer and far more effective at strengthening the abdominal muscles. Simply roll the head and shoulders up and forward and then roll back. The back stays flat to the floor and abdominal muscles should be pulled in.

>>: Straight leg lifts with both legs while lying on your back. This is extremely harmful to the back. It is okay to do one leg at a time if your hands are flat on the floor next to your hips helping to anchor your body.

>>: Standing toe touches either with the knees straight or bent. The toe touch is an excellent test of back and hamstring flexibility but only a test.

>>: Any bouncy movements.

>>: Anything that causes your back to arch.

CHAPTER   12
BEYOND   BACKHAB
A WATER WALKING PROGRAM

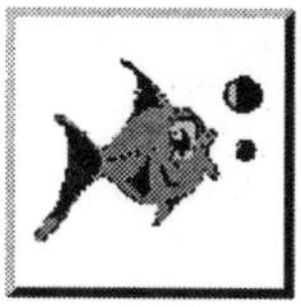

I f you're pain free and ready for an all
around safe, effective workout, it's time
to try the Aquawalk program. Shoes are
recommended.

THERMAL WARM UP
Do exercises A through G for 45 seconds
each.

A   Walk with small steps forward 12 and
    back 12 with walking arms (right arm
    swings forward as left leg steps
    forward) and elbows bent.
B   Repeat letter A with shoulder rolls.
C   Walk in a circle rolling from heel to toe.
D   Walk backward in circle rolling from
    toe to heel.
E   Walk around the circle on toes. (FIGURE 1)
F   Walk backwards around the circle on
    heels. (FIGURE 2)
G   Do ankle circles for 20 seconds with
    the right foot and 20 seconds with the
    left. (FIGURE 3)

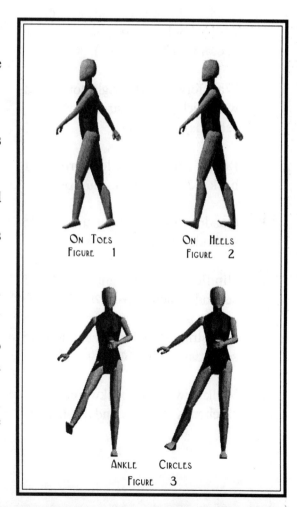

ON TOES
FIGURE   1

ON   HEELS
FIGURE   2

ANKLE   CIRCLES
FIGURE   3

PRE-STRETCH

A   Calf stretch right and left (15 seconds each). (FIGURE 4)

B   Walk forward around circle, push both arms forward for trapezius/rhomboid stretch (20 seconds). (FIGURE   5)

C   Walk backwards around the circle with a shoulder blade pinch to stretch pectorals (20 seconds). (FIGURE 6)

D   Walk forward to the right corner and walk back with hamstring curls (20 seconds). (FIGURE 7)

E   Repeat letter D to the left corner and back (20 seconds). (SEE FIGURE 7)

F   Quadricep stretch right and left (15 seconds each). (FIGURE 8)

G   Hip flexor stretch right and left (15 seconds each). (FIGURE 9)

H   Hamstring stretch right and left (15 seconds each). (FIGURE 10)

I   Walk forward and backwards with sidebends (30 seconds). (FIGURE 11)

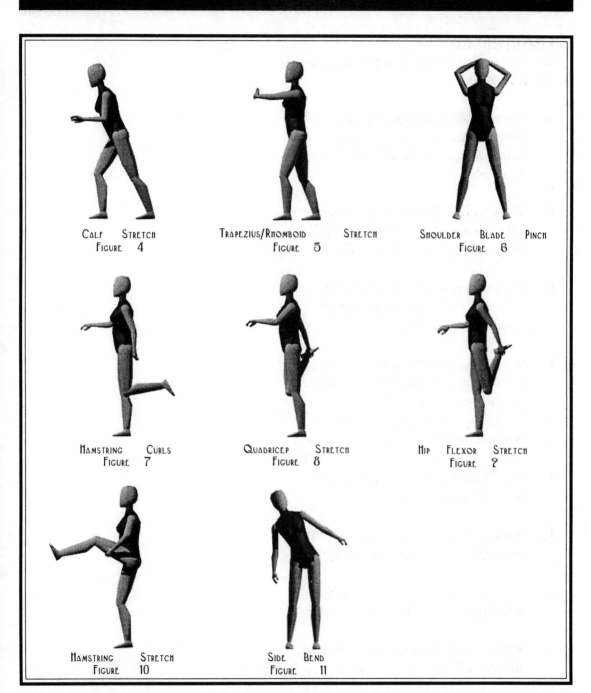

CALF   STRETCH
FIGURE 4

TRAPEZIUS/RHOMBOID   STRETCH
FIGURE 5

SHOULDER   BLADE   PINCH
FIGURE 6

HAMSTRING   CURLS
FIGURE 7

QUADRICEP   STRETCH
FIGURE 8

HIP   FLEXOR   STRETCH
FIGURE 9

HAMSTRING   STRETCH
FIGURE 10

SIDE   BEND
FIGURE 11

CARDIO WARM UP

Do exercises A through I for 45 seconds each in circle formation.

A   Moving forward, take exaggerated long strides with knees bent. Keep knees bent, while using jogging arms with hands cupped. (FIGURE 12)

B   Keep knees bent and move double time with smaller steps. Change arms to punching. (FIGURE 13)

C   Repeat A and B backing up.

Face center of circle for exercises D through I.

D   Walk sideways with lateral arms. Move 8 to the right and 8 to the left until the time allotment is finished. (FIGURE 14)

E   Walk sideways with deltoid lift arms. Move 8 to the right and 8 to the left until the time allotment is finished. (FIGURE 15)

F   Walk into and out of the circle with front crawl and back stroke arms. (FIGURE 16)

G   Add high knees to letter F and continue.

H   Straighten legs to a goose step moving in and out of the circle. (FIGURE 17)

I   Repeat E, F, G, H

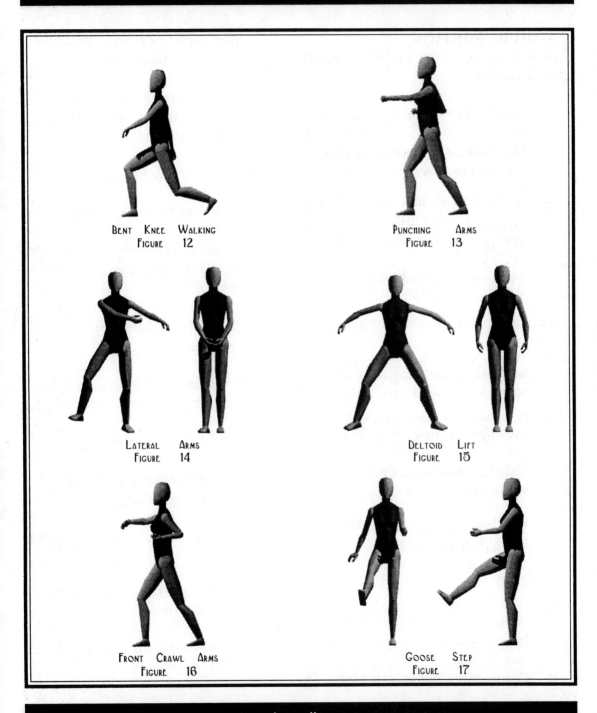

BENT KNEE WALKING
FIGURE   12

PUNCHING   ARMS
FIGURE   13

LATERAL   ARMS
FIGURE   14

DELTOID   LIFT
FIGURE   15

FRONT CRAWL ARMS
FIGURE   16

GOOSE   STEP
FIGURE   17

AEROBIC PORTION

Do the exercises below for 45-60 seconds each.

GROUP 1 *(facing forward)*

A   Walk forward on toes (bent elbow walking arms). Walk back on heels.

B   Walk sideways with a side kick. Move to the right 8 and 8 to the left until the time allotment is finished. (FIGURE 18)

C   Walk forward and back with hamstring curls. (SEE FIGURE 7, P.83)

GROUP 2

A   Walk in a square with knees and toes pointed somewhat out. (FIGURE 19)

B   Repeat letter A moving backwards with toes in. (FIGURE 20)

C   Walk forward and back with side bends. (SEE FIGURE 11, P.83)

D   Walk leaning forward moving forward, leaning back moving back.

GROUP 3

A   Walk forward into circle, with high knees.

B   Continue with high knees but cross

right foot over left and lower right as the step is taken. (FIGURE 21)

C   Walk backwards around the circle crossing the right foot behind the left and the left behind the right.

GROUP 4 *(in circle formation)*

A   Walk around the circle with high knees.

B   Continue walking around the circle but change to a goose step. (SEE FIGURE 17, P.85)

C   Same as B but change to a flick kick. (FIGURE 22)

D   Repeat letters A through C moving backwards around the circle.

GROUP 5

A   Walk around the circle, contracting and releasing abdominals.

B   Walk backwards with diagonal kicks. (FIGURE 23)

C   Side kick and step across moving forward. (FIGURE 24)

D   Side kick and step behind moving back.

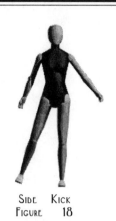

SIDE KICK
FIGURE 18

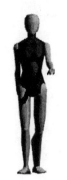

TOES OUT
FIGURE 19

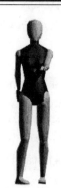

TOES IN
FIGURE 20

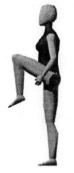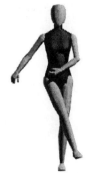

HIGH KNEE AND CROSS
FIGURE 21

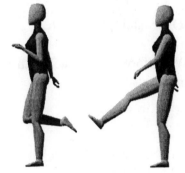

FLICK KICK
FIGURE 22

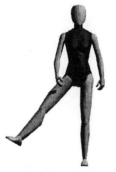

DIAGONAL KICK
FIGURE 23

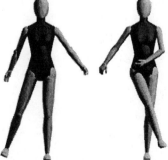

SIDE KICK AND STEP ACROSS
FIGURE 24

COOLDOWN

Do exercises A through E for one minute each *(face front)*.

A   Walk 4 low and 4 high - 2 sets moving forward and two sets moving back.
(FIGURE 25)

B   Walk 4 fast and 8 slow - forward and back.

C   Walk sideways 2 slow and 4 fast - 2 sets right, 2 sets left.

D   Over and present. (FIGURE 26)

E   Walk forward and back with shoulder rolls.

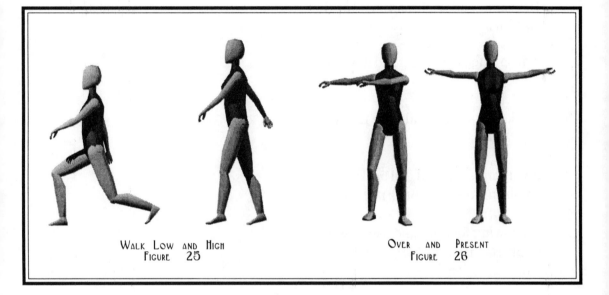

WALK LOW AND HIGH
FIGURE 25

OVER AND PRESENT
FIGURE 26

TONING SEGMENT *at pool edge*

Do each exercise for 24 repetitions or one minute. Those repeated on the right and left sides last for two minutes total.

A   Bicep curls right and then left. (FIGURE 27)

B   Hamstring curls right and then left. (SEE FIGURE 7, P.83)

C   Tricep extensions right and then left. (FIGURE 28)

D   Flick kicks right and then left. (SEE FIGURE 22, P.87)

E   Swing arms forward and back (with emphasis on pull back). (FIGURE 29)

F   Kickswing forward and back (with emphasis on pull back) right and then left. (FIGURE 30)

G   Deltoid lift (both arms at the same time). (SEE FIGURE 15, P.85)

H   Side lifts (hip abduction) right and then left. (FIGURE 31)

I   Press down (both arms at the same time). (FIGURE 32)

TONING SEGMENT CONTINUED ON PAGE 22 . . . .

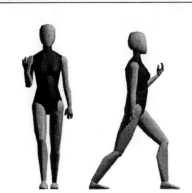

BICEP CURLS
FIGURE 27

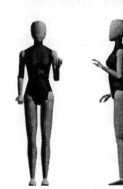

TRICEP EXTENSIONS
FIGURE 28

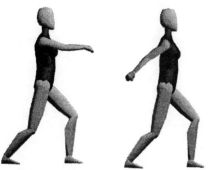

SWING ARMS FORWARD AND BACK
FIGURE 29

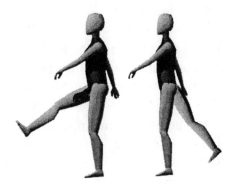

KICK SWING
FIGURE 30

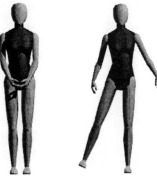

SIDE LIFTS
FIGURE 31

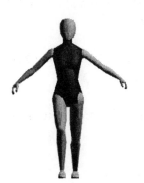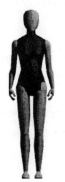

PRESS DOWN
FIGURE 32

CONTINUED FROM TONING SEGMENT ON PAGE 20

J   Cross kicks right and left. (FIGURE 33)

K   Elbow press forward.   (FIGURE 34)

L   Abdominal crunches.   (FIGURE 35)

M   Elbow press back.   (FIGURE 36)

N   Kick swing forward and back (with emphasis on the kick) right and then left. (SEE FIGURE 30, P. 21)

O   Swing arms forward and back (with emphasis on the swing forward). (SEE FIGURE 22, P. 21)

P   Punch across (alternating arms). (FIGURE 41)

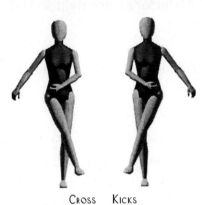
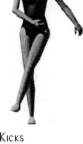

CROSS   KICKS
FIGURE   33

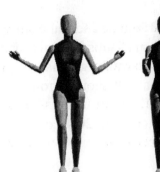
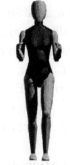
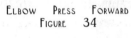

ELBOW   PRESS   FORWARD
FIGURE   34

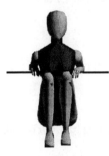
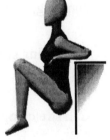
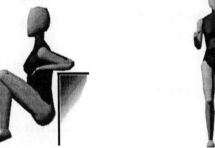

ABDOMINAL   CRUNCHES
FIGURE   35

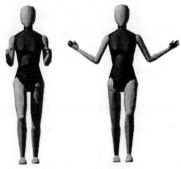

ELBOW   PRESS   BACK
FIGURE   36

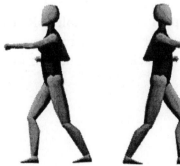

PUNCH   ACROSS
FIGURE   37

POSTSTRETCH

1. Do A and B from the Thermal Warmup. (Walk with small strps forward 12 and back 12 with walking arms, elbows bent. Repeat with shoulder rolls.)

2. Bicep stretch 15 to 20 seconds. (FIGURE 38)

3. Trapezius stretch 15 to 20 seconds. (FIGURE 3?)

4. Do C and D from the Thermal Warmup. (Walk in a circle rolling from heel to toe. Then walk backward in a circle rolling from toe to heel.)

5. Quadricep stretch right and left. (SEE FIGURE 8, P.83)

6. Hip flexor stretch right and left. (SEE FIGURE ?, P.83)

7. Do E from the Thermal Warmup (Walk around the circle on toes), with Tricep stretch right and left and Neck stretch right and left. (FIGURE 40)

8. Do F and G from the Thermal Warmup (Walk backwards around the circle on heels. Do ankle circles for 20 seconds with right foot and 20 seconds with the left.

9. Abductor stretch right and left. (FIGURE 41)

10. Adductor stretch right and left. (FIGURE 42)

11. Do A and B from Cardio Warmup (Moving forward, take exaggerated long strides with knees bent, while using jogging arms with hands cupped. Keep knees bent and move double time with smaller steps. Change arms to punching).

12. Hamstring stretch right and left. (SEE FIGURE 10, P.83)

13. Calf stretch right and left. (SEE FIGURE 4, P.83)

14. Back stretch. (FIGURE 43)

Back pain is preventable. Relearn the activities of daily living, exercise regularly, and enjoy good back health and comfort!

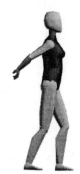

BICEP STRETCH
FIGURE 38

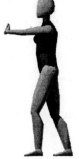

TRAPEZIUS STRETCH
FIGURE 39

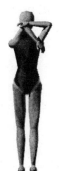 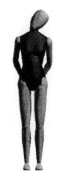

TRICEP STRETCH   NECK STRETCH
FIGURE 40

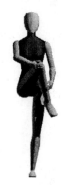

ABDUCTOR STRETCH
FIGURE 41

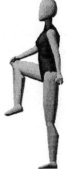

ADDUCTOR STRETCH
FIGURE 42

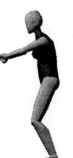 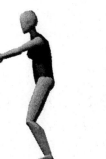

BACK STRETCH
FIGURE 43

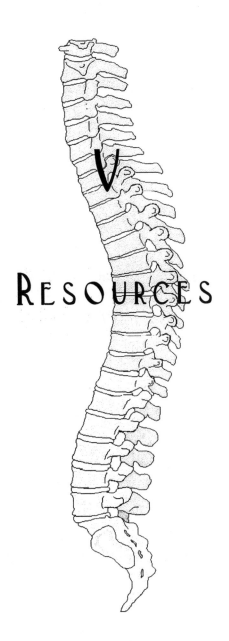

V

RESOURCES

CHAPTER 13

BACKLOG
BACKHAB PERSONAL RECORD

Prior to the start of the BackHab program, check with your therapist or doctor to make sure it's okay to begin the program. Take the book and show them the BackHab program and this log. They may want to modify it so that you would move faster or slower through the progression.

Week One

Sunday

 Fill out the pain questionnaire found in the Class Forms section of BackWords.

Monday

1. Do the Warm-up Walk and Alignment Work first. Take special care to feel comfortable in the water and with moving through the water with good upright alignment.

2. Do the Back Stretches and Abdominal Tightening section next. Keep them easy.

3. Repeat #1 and #2. They should feel a little easier to do the second time. You'll be more comfortable with the moves and you're body will be warmed up and wanting to try more.

 This workout will only take about 10 minutes today. You may want to do more but it's wise to wait to see how you feel after this much first.

 Write any comments about how you felt in the water, how the moves seemed, and how you felt afterwards.

_____

_____

_____

_____

_____

_____
_____
_____
_____
_____

Tuesday

🐟 Take note of how you feel today. You may not notice anything and that's good. That means you can go on to the next progression tomorrow. If you feel worse today than normal, you should repeat Monday's workout until it doesn't make you feel worse.

🐟 Write here if you noticed anything different today.

_____
_____
_____
_____
_____

🐟 Always work to the point to tension, not pain, when you're stretching. You should feel the effort but it shouldn't be painful.

Wednesday

1. Do the Warm-up Walk and Alignment Work first. Take special care to feel comfortable in the water and with moving through it with good upright alignment.

2. Do the Back Stretches and Abdominal Tightening section next. Keep them easy. Remember yesterday's note about stretching only to the point of tension.

3. Do the Alignment and Abdominal Work. Don't forget that there are two types of walking in the alignment work.

4. Repeat #1 and #2. They should be starting to become familiar now.

🐟 Write in the log today how the workout went. Did you have any problems with the wall stretches? If so, modify them and do the closest thing you can to copy them. Do only as much as is comfortable. Write here what you noticed.

_____
_____
_____
_____
_____
_____

today any new pain or any problems you may
have noticed after yesterday's workout.
Write here about how you feel today.

_____
_____
_____
_____
_____
_____

📌 If you had problems walking with the forceful abdominal contractions try to stand and do them next time. Simply stand in the water, think about the sponge in your stomach, and try to squeeze it out by using the abdominal muscles. Don't do too many in a row while you're standing still. The program calls for three steps between "crunches" to protect you from doing too much and to continue the strengthening you'll get from walking.

Thursday

📌 Follow the progression tomorrow only if you feel no new problems today. Notice

📌 Remember the two hour pain rule. If you have more pain two hours after exercising than when you began you probably tried to do too much. Do less during the next workout.

Friday

📌 If you had no new problems after Wednesday's workout, do the following workout today.

1. Do the Warm-up Walk and Alignment Work first. Take special

care to feel comfortable in the water and with moving through it with good upright alignment.

2. Do the Back Stretches and Abdominal Tightening section next. Keep them easy.

3. Do the Alignment and Abdominal Work. Remember, there are two types of walking in the alignment work. You'll do a regular align ment walk first and then do the abdominal contraction walk. If you have problems with this refer back to Wednesday's log to review suggestions on how it might work for you.

4. Do the High Knee Walking. This is a difficult progression because it's quite exertive. Do what you can while remembering to keep the spine upright during the lift of the knee and during the press down when the knee straightens. That way whatever you do will be safe, no matter how much or little it is. Try not to do too much. This is one you may really feel later. If it feels difficult to you, don't move forward or back. Stay in one place and lift your knee easily and press it down slowly.

5. Repeat #1 and #2. They should be starting to become easy to remember

and do now.

 Enter in your log today how you felt during the workout, if any move felt particularly good or bothered you, and how you felt after the workout.

_____

_____

_____

_____

_____

_____

_____

_____

_____

Saturday

 How do you feel today? Did you keep yesterday's stretches to only light tension? All stretching, even for well conditioned athletes, should be held easily with light tension. Don't push your stretches. Take it easy.

 Write today about your pain. Do you

hurt more, less or the same? List any changes in the location of your pain, the type of pain, or what you do that creates more pain.

_____

_____

_____

_____

_____

_____

Week Two

Sunday

🐟 Read the preface of this book today and remind yourself to stay on track but, even more importantly, to stay light hearted and enjoy yourself.

🐟 Again write about your pain today. Notice different activities that create immediate pain and others that you think contribute to your chronic pain.

_____

_____

_____

_____

_____

_____

Monday

🐟 If you had no new problems after Friday's workout, do the following workout today.

1. Do the Warm-up Walk and Alignment Work first. Always take special care to get comfortable in the water and enjoy moving through it with good upright alignment.

2. Do the Back Stretches and Abdominal Tightening section next. Keep them easy.

3. Do the Alignment and Abdominal Work. Remember, there are two types of walking in the alignment work. You'll do a regular alignment walk first and then do the abdominal contraction walk. If you have problems with this refer back to last Wednesday's

log to review suggestions on how it might work for you.

4. Do the High Knee Walking. This is a difficult progression because it's quite exertive. It's fine to stay in place. You can start by doing several kneelifts in place before moving forward and backwards. Keep the spine upright during the lift of the knee and during the press down when the knee straightens. That way whatever you do will be safe, no matter how much or little it is. Try not to do too much. This is one you may really feel later.

5. Do the Back Stretches and Abdominal Tightening again. Concentrate on pulling your stomach in, and rounding or flattening your back on all the exercises.

6. Do the Alignment and Abdominal Work again. Always remember to move backwards as well as forwards. The backward moving exercises are excellent in creating muscle balance for us. We're very comfortable with moving forward but the muscles that move us backwards rarely get used. Give the backward moving time some extra effort today. Most importantly, walk tall and picture yourself strong,

fit and healthy.

7. Do the High Knee Walking again. It's exertive so you must move slowly. The muscles that help you push your leg down (after the kneelift) need to do the work. If you move too quickly or you're not in good alignment, the back muscles will have to do the job. We already have them working on other things so let's not use them here. If you're moving forward and backwards, remember that you don't need to move very far on each step.

5. Repeat #1 and #2. They're like old friends now!

It's time to write. You know the drill.

_____

_____

_____

_____

_____

_____

_____

_____

_____

Tuesday

How do you feel today? Do you feel any changes? Your workout yesterday was longer and quite exertive. If you or your muscles feel weak today you may want to repeat yesterday's workout tomorrow and put off tomorrow's workout for awhile. Tomorrow's workout will be easier in terms of length and stamina, but more difficult on the leg muscles. Write about how you feel today.

_____

_____

_____

_____

_____

How was your water depth yesterday? If you weren't sure of the water you probably started the program last week in waist depth water. If you're more comfortable now you can move a little deeper. Midriff depth seems

best for most people. Try it tomorrow and see how it works for you.

Wednesday

1. Do the Warm-up Walk and Alignment Work first. Always take special care to get comfortable in the water and enjoy moving through it with good upright alignment.

2. Do the Back Stretches and Abdominal Tightening section next. Concentrate on pulling your stomach in, and rounding or flattening your back on all the exercises. Keep them easy.

3. Do the Alignment and Abdominal Work. Give the backward moving time some extra effort again today. Walk tall and picture yourself strong, fit and healthy.

4. Do the High Knee Walking. You can start by doing several kneelifts in place before moving forward and backwards. Keep the spine upright during the lift of the knee and during the press down when the knee straightens. This is exertive so you must move slowly. You don't need to move very far on each step.

5. Do the Long Stride Walking while staying tall like you have been with the other walking. Sometimes lengthening the stride challenges our balance so much that we lean forward. Keep reminding yourself to lift your ribs. This walk will do wonderful things for you if you let it.

6. Repeat #1 and #2. They're like old friends now!

Are the wall stretches getting easier? Write down what's working and what doesn't feel right. Also, take note of how your pain feels when you're in the pool. Sometimes you'll start to be pain-free when you're in the water long before you're pain-free out of the water.

_____

_____

_____

_____

_____

_____

_____

_____

_____

Thursday

Did you wake up with any new pain today? Take note, and write down, how you feel. The Long Stride Walking stretched your muscles in new ways yesterday.

_____

_____

_____

_____

_____

How has the water temperature felt for you? It should be warm enough. If it isn't, you may be stiffening up and creating more tension and pain. If that's happening, look in the Resource section of BackWords in this book for D.K. Douglas and call them for a catalog. They make vests and pants that keep you warm in the water. When you're too cold all your blood gets shunted to the vital organs. That leaves your arms and legs cold. The vest keeps your vital organs warm so the blood can move to your extremities and warm your arms and legs.

Friday

If you've experienced no new problems this week do the following workout.

1. Do the Warm-up Walk and Alignment Work first. Don't skip this section in your haste to get to the "real" work. This part is here to get your body ready for the "real" work. If your body isn't ready, you could create more pain and problems for yourself.

2. Do the Back Stretches and Abdominal Tightening section next. Concentrate on pulling your stomach in, and rounding or flattening your back on all the exercises. Keep them easy and hold them for the full counts.

3. Do the Alignment and Abdominal Work. Give the backward moving time some extra effort again today. Walk tall and picture yourself strong, fit and healthy. Visualizations work.

4. Do the High Knee Walking. Keep the spine upright during the lift of the

knee and during the press down when the knee straightens. This is exertive so you must move slowly.

5. Do the Long Stride Walking while staying tall like you have been with the other walking. Sometimes lengthening the stride challenges our balance so much that we lean forward. Keep reminding yourself to lift your ribs.

6. Do the Back Stretches and Abdominal Tightening again. These exercises are the core of the BackHab program. You can do them between each walking exercise if you like. They gently work on the muscle imbalance between the back and stomach muscles.

7. Do the Alignment and Abdominal Work again. Now that you're comfortable with the walking you might want to think about covering more territory with each step. Start to challenge yourself and your trunk muscles. If you start to lose alignment, shorten the stride a little.

8. Do the High Knee Walking again. When backing up be sure to lift your knee as high as you can in front of you. That will doubly challenge the

gluteal muscles that need to push your knee down to step back. If you feel any of the work radiating into the low back, slow down.

9. Do the Long Stride Walking again. This time think about stepping forward with your heel. Make sure the heel touches first as you step forward. The back leg should be pushing off with the toes.

10. Repeat #1 and #2.

This workout was a big jump in time. Did it work okay for you? Write about the workout today.

_____

_____

_____

_____

_____

_____

_____

Be sure to keep the exercises feeling like they're so easy they couldn't possibly work. That way you'll have fun with a simple workout and your body will respond by getting stronger without you even knowing it.

Saturday

Chart your pain symptoms today.

_____

_____

_____

_____

_____

Reread Chapter 5 on home treating your back problems. Be sure you have a home treatable back!

Week Three

Sunday

Today think about your alignment as you

go through your regular schedule. List one thing that you could change easily.

_____

_____

_____

_____

Monday

Do this workout only if you had no problems with Friday's workout. It's exactly the same as Friday's workout except we're adding the Cooldown and Final Stretches.

1. Do the Warm-up Walk and Alignment Work first. Don't skip this section in your haste to get to the "real" work. This part is here to get your body ready for the "real" work. If your body isn't ready, you could create more pain and problems for yourself.

2. Do the Back Stretches and Abdominal Tightening section next. Concentrate on pulling your stomach in, and rounding or flattening your back on all the exercises. Keep them easy and hold them for the full counts.

3. Do the Alignment and Abdominal Work. Give the backward moving time some extra effort again today. Walk tall and picture yourself strong, fit and healthy. Visualizations work.

4. Do the High Knee Walking. Keep the spine upright during the lift of the knee and during the press down when the knee straightens. This is exertive so you must move slowly.

5. Do the Long Stride Walking while staying tall like you have been with the other walking. Sometimes lengthening the stride challenges our balance so much that we lean forward. Keep reminding yourself to lift your ribs.

6. Do the Back Stretches and Abdominal Tightening again. These exercises are the core of the BackHab program. You can do them between each walking exercise if you like. They gently work on the muscle imbalance between the back and stomach muscles.

7. Do the Alignment and Abdominal Work again. Now that you're comfortable with the walking you might want to think about covering more territory with each step. Start to challenge yourself and your trunk muscles. If you start to lose

alignment, shorten the stride a little.
8. Do the High Knee Walking again.
When backing up be sure to lift your
knee as high as you can in front of
you. That will doubly challenge the
gluteal muscles that need to push your
knee down to step back. If you feel
any of the work radiating into the low
back, slow down.

9. Do the Long Stride Walking again.
This time think about stepping
forward with your heel. Make sure
the heel touches first as you step
forward. The back leg should be
pushing off with the toes.

10. Do the Cooldown and Final
Stretches. These are some new
stretches. Review them and do the
segment twice. Do them easily and
in whatever way works best for you.

 It's time to write!

_____

_____

_____

_____

_____

Tuesday

 How do you feel today? You've been
putting in heavy workouts. Track changes
that you're noticing. If any of those changes
include additional pain cut back immediately
on the workout. Go back to week two or the
point where you didn't experience additional
pain. Gradually build up after that.

_____

_____

_____

_____

_____

 Are you using shoes? You should be

wearing shoes during the BackHab program to protect yourself from slipping on the deck or pool bottom. Check the Resources section of BackWords and order catalogs from HydroFit, Sprint Rothhammer and Ryka.

Wednesday

If you had no problems with Monday's workout, let's try adding some Power work!

1. Do the Warm-up Walk and Alignment Work first.

2. Do the Back Stretches and Abdominal Tightening section next. These exercises are the core of the BackHab program. You can do them between each walking exercise if you like. They gently work on the muscle imbalance between the back and stomach muscles.

3. Do the Alignment and Abdominal Work. Walk tall and picture yourself strong, fit and healthy. Visualizations work. Now that you're comfortable with the walking you might want to think about covering more territory with each step. Start to challenge yourself and your trunk muscles. If you start to lose alignment, shorten the stride a little.

4. Do the High Knee Walking. When backing up be sure to lift your knee as high as you can in front of you. That will doubly challenge the gluteal muscles that need to push your knee down to step back. If you feel any of the work radiating into the low back, slow down.

5. Do the Long Stride Walking. This time think about stepping forward with your heel. Make sure the heel touches first as you step forward. The back leg should be pushing off with the toes. Keep reminding yourself to lift your ribs.

6. Do the Power Walking. Follow the directions moving slowly and keeping your torso upright.

7. Do the Cooldown and Final Stretches. Review them and do the stretches segment twice. Do them easily and in whatever way works best for you.

You worked your legs hard today. How did the workout feel? What was great and what was uncomfortable? How was your pain in the pool? Log everything you can think of.

_____

_____

_____

_____

_____

🐟 Be sure to stay upright during the power walk and let your legs do the work.

Thursday

🐟 Continue to watch yourself for changing patterns in your pain. Maybe the pain is in a new location, maybe it's dull instead of numbing, or sharp instead of boring. Write those things down. Also write about how your feel during the BackHab workout.

_____

_____

_____

_____

_____

_____

_____

Friday

🐟 If you had no problems with Wednesday's workout, give this one a try.

1. Do the Warm-up Walk and Alignment Work first.

2. Do the Back Stretches and Abdominal Tightening section next. These exercises are the core of the BackHab program. You can do them between each walking exercise if you like. They gently work on the muscle imbalance between the back and stomach muscles.

3. Do the Alignment and Abdominal Work. Walk tall and picture yourself strong, fit and healthy. Visualizations work. Now that you're comfortable with the walking you might want to think about covering more territory with each step. Start to challenge yourself and your trunk muscles. If you start to lose alignment, shorten the stride a little.

4. Do the High Knee Walking. When backing up be sure to lift your knee as

high as you can in front of you. That will doubly challenge the gluteal muscles that need to push it down to step back. If you feel any of the work radiating into the low back, slow down.

5. Do the Long Stride Walking. Keep reminding yourself to lift your ribs.

6. Do the Power Walking. Follow the directions moving slowly and keeping your torso upright.

5. Do the Long Stride Walking again. This time think about stepping forward with your heel. Make sure the heel touches first as you step forward. The back leg should be pushing off with the toes. Keep reminding yourself to lift your ribs.

6. Do the Power Walking again. This is a tough one and a very powerful workout for your legs. By moving through the water all your trunk muscles get a workout too. Move slowly and keep your torso upright.

7. Do the Cooldown and Final Stretches. Review them and do the stretches segment twice again today. Continue to do them easily and in whatever way works best for you.

Your workouts are getting more demanding. Write about anything you noticed today.

_____

_____

_____

_____

_____

_____

_____

_____

If you become exhausted or your muscles feel weak and shaky, you should do less. If you became energized, continue to follow the progression.

Saturday

Write again about how you're feeling today.

_____

_____

_____

_____

_____

_____

_____

🐟: Reread Chapter 8, An Ounce of Prevention, and start to think about implementing one prevention technique in your life.

Week Four

Sunday

🐟: Notice how you feel today, your second day in a row of no BackHab.

_____

_____

_____

_____

_____

🐟: If you feel better from the BackHab program add an extra very light day of it if you want this week.

Monday

🐟: Follow this progression if you've been feeling fine with the BackHab program. It's a double them up, review day.

1. Do the Warm-up Walk and Alignment Work first.

2. Do the Back Stretches and Abdominal Tightening section next. These exercises are the core of the BackHab program. You can do them between each walking exercise if you like. They gently work on the muscle imbalance between the back and stomach muscles.

3. Do the Alignment and Abdominal Work.

4. Do the High Knee Walking.

5. Do the Long Stride Walking. Keep reminding yourself to lift your ribs.

6. Do the Power Walking.

7. Do the Alignment and Abdominal work again. Now that you're comfortable with the walking you might want to think about covering more territory with each step. Start to challenge yourself and your trunk

muscles. If you start to lose alignment, shorten the stride a little.

8. Do the High Knee Walking again. When backing up be sure to lift your knee as high as you can in front of you. That will doubly challenge the gluteal muscles that need to push your knee down to step back. If you feel any of the work radiating into the low back, slow down.

9. Do the Long Stride Walking again. This time think about stepping forward with your heel. Make sure the heel touches first as you step forward. The back leg should be pushing off with the toes. Keep reminding yourself to lift your ribs.

10. Do the Power Walking again. This is a tough one and a very powerful workout for your legs. By moving through the water all your trunk muscles get a workout too. Move slowly and keep your torso upright.

11. Do the Cooldown and Final Stretches. Do the stretches once. Continue to do them easily and in whatever way works best for you.

 This is a long workout! Be sure to

record how you feel while you're doing it and how you feel afterwards.

_____

_____

_____

_____

_____

_____

_____

_____

_____

_____

 On Wednesday we'll start adding new moves again.

Tuesday

 Remember alignment when registering how you're feeling today. Were you able to keep good alignment during the BackHab workout yesterday? If not, you may want to repeat it until you feel better about it. Write about the workout and how you're doing.

_____

_____
_____
_____
_____

🐟 If you need alignment reminders think about letting your shoulders relax and drop comfortably and about lifting your ribs. We want the lungs to be able to get oxygen to the muscles so you can strengthen the muscles. If you lift your ribs the lungs won't be squeezed and they'll be able to work well for you. Congratulations! You're progressing.

Wednesday

🐟 If you had no problems with Monday's workout, let's try adding some oblique work!

1. Do the Warm-up Walk and Alignment Work first.

2. Do the Back Stretches and Abdominal Tightening section next. You can do them between each walking exercise if you like.

3. Do the Alignment and Abdominal Work. Walk tall.

4. Do the High Knee Walking.

5. Do the Long Stride Walking.

6. Do the Power Walking.

7. Do the Oblique Abdominal Muscles first exercise only (figure 10, p35). We'll do the sidelift and power dip on future days. Begin by simply putting one foot in front of the other and then progress to crossing them over each other. If you've had a hip replacement do not do this exercise unless you clear it with your physician or therapist.

8. Do the Cooldown and Final Stretches.

🐟 It's time to record how the workout felt. Go for it.

_____
_____
_____
_____

_____

_____

_____

🐟: We're starting to actively involve the midriff muscles. When you cross over with your legs during the new exercise try to keep your shoulders forward. That will get the obliques and quadratus lumborum working.

Thursday

🐟: How do you feel today? Did the midriff work set off any problems? If so, you know to go back and ease into yesterday's workout more lightly.

_____

_____

_____

_____

_____

_____

🐟: Tension, not pain. Not only the stretches but also the exercises should be done with this guideline in mind. Working out should be easy and fun. This is not the time to think about adding equipment. If you're feeling strong do a little extra walking at the pool tomorrow.

Friday

🐟: Take stock before you jump in today. Are you ready for more or should you repeat the last workout a few times before moving forward. If you're ready, here's the workout.

1. Do the Warm-up Walk and Alignment Work.

2. Do the Back Stretches and Abdominal Tightening section. You can do them between each walking exercise if you like.

3. Do the Alignment and Abdominal Work.

4. Do the High Knee Walking.

5. Do the Long Stride Walking.

6. Do the Power Walking.

7. Do the Oblique Abdominal Muscles first exercise (figure 10. p.35). Begin by simply putting one foot in front of the

other and then progress to crossing them over each other. If you've had a hip replacement do not do this exercise unless you clear it with your physician or therapist.

8. Do the Oblique Abdominal Muscles second exercise (figure 11, p35). Again, if you've had a hip replacement do not do this exercise unless you clear it with your physician or therapist. Pullthe leg down easily from the out position.

9. Do the Cooldown and Final Stretches.

🐟 How did it feel? Write even things that you think aren't important.

_____

_____

_____

_____

_____

_____

_____

_____

_____
_____

🐟 When doing the sidelift during the second oblique exercise try to keep your toe pointed forward, not out. This will ensure use of the abductors rather than the hip flexors. Be gentle when lowering your leg from the sidelift. Using force could cause back problems. You can be more exertive on this exercise when you're ready for the Water Walking program.

Saturday

🐟 Reread Chapter 6, Rules Rules Rules, to make sure you're following all the guidelines.

<u>Week Five</u>

Sunday

🐟 Take today to rest your back. When you move around notice what activities increase, decrease or change your pain. Write those down along with how you're feeling today.

_____

_____

_____

_____

_____

_____

_____

Monday

🐟: Take stock again before you jump in today. Are you ready for more or should you repeat the last workout a few times before moving forward. If you're ready, here's the workout.

1. Do the Warm-up Walk and Alignment Work.

2. Do the Back Stretches and Abdominal Tightening section. You can do them between each walking exercise if you like.

3. Do the Alignment and Abdominal Work.

4. Do the High Knee Walking.

5. Do the Long Stride Walking.

6. Do the Power Walking.

7. Do the Oblique Abdominal Muscles first exercise (figure 10, p35). Begin by simply putting one foot in front of the other and then progress to crossing them over each other. If you've had a hip replacement do not do this exercise unless you clear it with your physician or therapist.

8. Do the Oblique Abdominal Muscles second exercise (figure 11, p35). Again, if you've had a hip replacement do not do this exercise unless you clear it with your physician or therapist. Pull the leg down easily from the out position.

9. Do the Oblique Abominal Muscles third exercise (figure 12, p35). Once more, if you've had a hip replacement do not do this exercise unless you clear it with your physician or therapist. Get all your weight over the leg that's going to push you up. The other leg will simply lift out to the side as it did in the last exercise.

10. Do the Cooldown and Final Stretches.

🐟: How did that feel? If you've gotten this far you're doing really well. This was

very exertive. Write notes on how you felt
during the workout and afterwards. Be sure
to mention any changes in your pain.

_____

_____

_____

_____

_____

_____

_____

_____

🐟 During our next workout we'll be
moving side to side, not forward and
backwards. It should make the next three
additions fairly easy for you to do.

Tuesday

🐟 Log how you feel today. You've added
some very difficult moves.

_____

_____

_____

_____

_____

_____

_____

🐟 Check the water depth you've been
using again. Is it at midriff? Are you able to
move with control? If you're too "floaty"
move a little shallower.

Wednesday

🐟 Are you ready? You know your body
best. Listen to your body and let it tell you
when you need to rest and when you can
continue.

1. Do the Warm-up Walk and
Alignment Work.

2. Do the Back Stretches and
Abdominal Tightening section. You
can do them between each walking
exercise if you like.

3. Do the Alignment and Abdominal Work.

_____

_____

4. Do the High Knee Walking.

_____

5. Do the Long Stride Walking.

_____

6. Do the Power Walking.

_____

7. Do the Oblique Abdominal Muscles. Do all three exercises, but remember, if you've had a hip replacement do not do this exercise unless you clear it with your physician or therapist.

8. Do the Thighs and Isometric Abdominal Work first exercise. Simply step sideways while thinking about your alignment.

9. Do the Cooldown and Final Stretches.

🐟 Chart how you feel today. List everything you can think of.

_____

_____

_____

_____

_____

🐟 When doing the sidestep begin easily and gradually increase the width of the stride.

Thursday

🐟 Log in how you feel again today. You used different muscles yesterday and will use them more during the next two workouts.

_____

_____

_____

_____

_____

_____

_____

🐟 We're working toward full muscle balance now. You're doing good!

Friday

🐟 If you're ready for a little more sidestepping, here it is.

1. Do the Warm-up Walk and Alignment Work.

2. Do the Back Stretches and Abdominal Tightening section. It is beneficial for you to do them between each walking exercise.

3. Do the Alignment and Abdominal Work.

4. Do the High Knee Walking.

5. Do the Long Stride Walking.

6. Do the Power Walking.

7. Do the Oblique Abdominal Muscles. Do all three exercises, but remember, if you've had a hip replacement do not do this exercise unless you clear it with your physician or therapist.

8. Do the Thighs and Isometric Abdominal Work first exercise. Simply step sideways while thinking about your alignment.

9. Do the Thighs and Isometric Abdominal Work second exercise (figure 13). Begin with the power dip only and then add the abdominal contractions. Again if you have trouble with the contractions, stay in place and do them rather than moving.

10. Do the Cooldown and Final Stretches.

🐟 Time to write how you feel today. The power work has a very high energy cost. Don't feel disappointed if you're tired out today.

_____
_____
_____
_____
_____
_____
_____
_____

Your thighs got a great workout today. Your back should feel good. Don't bend too much on the dip. If you bend too much you may start to use back muscles. Keep your spine straight.

Saturday

Look through the deep water exercises in Chapter 7 and decide if you'll be trying them. If so, check at your pool or in the Resource section for flotation equipment.

Log in about how you feel today.

_____

_____

_____

_____

_____

_____

Week Six

Sunday

Last week you used some new muscles in powerful ways. Today may be a great rest day. This week we'll add the final progressions. In the meantime, how do you feel today?

_____

_____

_____

_____

_____

Monday

If your body says "okay", here's the workout.

1. Do the Warm-up Walk and Alignment Work.

2. Do the Back Stretches and Abdominal Tightening section. It is

beneficial for you to do them between each walking exercise.

3. Do the Alignment and Abdominal Work.

4. Do the High Knee Walking.

5. Do the Long Stride Walking.

6. Do the Power Walking.

7. Do the Oblique Abdominal Muscles. Do all three exercises, but remember, if you've had a hip replacement do not do this exercise unless you clear it with your physician or therapist.

8. Do the Thighs and Isometric Abdominal Work first exercise. Simply step sideways while thinking about your alignment.

9. Do the Thighs and Isometric Abdominal Work second exercise (figure 13). Begin with the power dip only and then add the abdominal contractions. Again if you have trouble with the contractions, stay in place and do them rather than moving.

10. Do the Thighs and Isometric Abdominal Work third exercise (figure 14). Do not do this exercise

if you've had a hip replacement unless you clear it with your physician or therapist. This exercise isn't as difficult for the muscles as it is for your balance and coordination!

11. Do the Cooldown and Final Stretches.

You made it through another workout. How do you feel? How did it feel?

_____

_____

_____

_____

_____

_____

_____

_____

New pain during your workout means stop. If you feel new pain while doing BackHab, stop the exercise you're doing and move to one that doesn't create pain.

Tuesday

You know the routine. It's time to jot notes about how you're feeling.

_____

_____

_____

_____

_____

_____

_____

You're doing the whole shallow water program now. Continue to follow the program as you did yesterday unless you want to add the deep water progressions that follow.

Wednesday

If you're going to add the deep water work, here's the first workout with it included.

1. Do the Warm-up Walk and Alignment Work.

2. Do the Back Stretches and Abdominal Tightening section. It is beneficial for you to do them between each walking exercise.

3. Do the Alignment and Abdominal Work.

4. Do the High Knee Walking.

5. Do the Long Stride Walking.

6. Do the Power Walking.

7. Do the Oblique Abdominal Muscles. Do all three exercises, but remember, if you've had a hip replacement do not do this exercise unless you clear it with your physician or therapist.

8. Do the Thighs and Isometric Abdominal Work but do not do the crossover if you've had a hip replacement unless you clear it with your physician or therapist.

9. Move to the deep water and do the Jog, High Knee Jog, and High Knee Jog with Abdominal Contractions. Stay upright and tall.

10. Do the Cooldown and Final Stretches.

How did the deep water feel? How do you feel?

_____

_____

_____

_____

_____

_____

_____

_____

_____

_____

_____

_____

You won't move far with the deep water work. That's not the purpose in any of the BackHab program. The purpose is to train the muscles to keep you upright in a position that's safe and, hopefully, pain-free.

Thursday

How do you feel today? Did the deep water work make any difference?

If you added deep exercises be sure to review how you feel today. Without the stabilizing pool bottom you may feel some new pain. If so, do fewer repetitions next time and keep the midriff strong.

Friday

This is it ... the final progression! Congratulations, you've worked hard and must care very much about improving yourself.

1. Do the Warm-up Walk and Alignment Work.

2. Do the Back Stretches and Abdominal Tightening section. It is beneficial for you to do them between each walking exercise.

3. Do the Alignment and Abdominal Work.

CHAPTER 14
BACKWORDS
APPENDIX AND BIBLIOGRAPHY

BackHab Question And Answer

Q: My back hurts but my attitude is good - does that help?

A: YES! Dr. Thomas McKeown, a prominent English physician, said, "It is now evident that the health of man is determined predominantly, not by medical intervention, but, by his behavior, his food, and the nature of the world in which he finds himself." Practicing muscular and mental relaxation techniques, visualization, self-responsibility, cognitive concepts, imagery and positive affirmations will all help in gaining overall fitness. The mind-body connection in overall fitness and overall sickness works. The emotionally stable person with a positive attitude will be less likely to suffer from physical diseases.

There is not only a psychological phenomenon that improves the mental attitude of the regular exerciser but also a physical one. While the exact effects of powerful hormones called endorphins are not clear yet, they seem to be related to pain, emotions, the immune system, exercise and the reproduction system. The feelings of well-being that come with vigorous exercise have been traced to endorphins. They may also have an effect on mental problems. Patients with depression often have low levels of endorphins.

Q: I feel more alert and smarter after I do the water walking program. Is that just my self esteem?

A: The mind-body connection also correlates with mental sharpness, alertness and, sometimes, intelligence. A study at Purdue University found that after working out three times a week for six months, one group was not only 20% fitter, they scored 70% better in a test of complex decision making.

Q: Sometimes my eyes feel sensitive after my BackHab program even though I haven't put my face in the water. What's up?

A: We all know about using a sun block for our skin but many don't know that the sunlight can hurt our eyes just like skin. Not only does the sunshine present a problem for many aquatic exercisers but the water we're working in creates more. The glare from the reflective water (yes, even in indoor pools) and the chlorine increase the possibility of problems.

Q: What will happen?

A: You can get eye burn from the sun's reflection off the water. The IR (infrared) light rays cause eye fatigue and accelerate the effect of the UV (ultra violet) rays. Prolonged UV light exposure causes inflammation of the cornea and can lead to the development of cataracts.

Q: What's the solution?

Hats, visors, glasses and the football players' black streak under the eyes! Glasses which can cost $7 to $200 should offer good vision (not distort or dampen visual contrast) and still protect our eyes.

Polarized, brown contrast, lightweight wraparounds seem best. Double radiant filters are good too. The glasses should offer good depth perception, be lightweight and provide space for ventilation.

Here are some terms that might help:

Polarized means that the lenses will eliminate reflective glare from the large amounts of light hitting water. Polarized lenses are best against the glare of the water and they block the UV rays.

Gradient means that the lens is darker at the top than the bottom. They're not ideal for water but they're good protection from overhead sun. Unless they're also polarized they don't block the UV rays.

Double gradient means that the lens is darker at the top and at the bottom but clear in the middle. They're better for the water but not so good if the sun is directly in the horizon. Unless they're also polarized, they don't block the UV rays.

Flash reflective lenses have a mirror-like finish of silver, blue, rose or green. They reflect the light away instead of absorbing it like the other lenses.

Sports shields are usually wrap around and shield the eyes from above, below and the sides. They are made to protect the eyes from water, sweat, hair, dust and debris. They may help lessen the exposure to chlorine. These are the culprits behind the funny looking "raccoon eye" sun tans!

Cosmetic lenses are usually lightly tinted. They're generally not for pools because they don't offer enough protection.

General purpose lenses are usually medium to dark tint. They're not good enough for aquatics unless they're used exclusively inside with the only sunshine exposure through windows.

High index, *polycarbonate* and *UV tinted lenses* block 99% of UV rays, offer maximum protection, and are considered best for aquatics.

Q: My friend has back problems and fibromyalgia. I understand back problems, I don't understand fibromyalgia.

A: Millions of people have fibromyalgia. This is a fairly new term and new medical diagnosis, and therefore may be new to all of us. What is it and what can be done to cope with it?

Fibromyalgia is a disease in which muscles ache nonstop. People with the disease experience muscle pain all over, they are tired most of the time, they're afraid to get involved in anything physical including exercise, and they sleep poorly.

Fibromyalgia mostly affects middle aged women. Ninety percent of all patients are female and aged just under 50. The disease is uncommon in children and the elderly. No cure exists for fibromyalgia. Doctor's are only able to make suggestions to relieve the painful symptoms. Their recommendations usually include taking warm baths; applying heat; massage; following a regular sleep schedule; sleeping 8 hours a night; avoiding alcohol, caffeine and tobacco before bedtime; taking mid-day naps if possible; using relaxation techniques; and surprisingly, exercise.

Q: Why exercise if they hurt?

A: Regular workouts contribute to a general sense of well being and help people with fibromyalgia become more fit, more flexible, have better blood flow to the painful muscles, and achieve better posture. If you or someone you know has fibromyalgia the most important things to remember when working out are "good posture" and "keep it easy".

Good posture. Maintain a good posture while working out. This will help to align the muscles and allow you to understand and use good body mechanics for daily activities. All movement throughout the day should involve good, upright posture. For example, stand up tall and sit tall. Go upstairs without leaning forward and without pulling yourself up with the railing.

Keep it easy. If you have fibromyalgia you should avoid muscle fatigue. The disease can be made worse by muscular fatigue. This is the reason most sufferers have stayed away from any type of exercise or activity. You could end up with more pain afterwards.

It's important to keep the exercise at a low intensity, with rest breaks if necessary, to reduce the possibility of muscular fatigue. Many people with fibromyalgia have found that low impact, low intensity aerobic exercise can markedly improve their symptoms.

People with the disease who begin an exercise program are usually fatigued, in pain, and in poor condition from inactivity. It's okay if they are only able to participate in a five minute warm-up when first beginning. From that small amount of activity, they can gradually progress one to three minutes a week. The intensity should not increase. Always stay at a low "walking" level. It's best to build up to 30 minutes of exercise three times a week.

Fibromyalgia seems frightening at first. Once we understand exactly what it is, what it's symptoms are, and what we can do to alleviate the symptoms, it's not so bad. Exercise can help...let it!

BackHab Quiz

1. Most back pain is caused by:

a. lifting incorrectly
b. muscle imbalance
c. osteoporosis
d. fat stomachs

2. How much of our population will have back problems at some time in their lives?

a. 80 to 85% of the population
b. 18 million
c. 25% of the population
d. 90% of the male population

3. Aquatic Exercise is ideal for people with back pain because:

a. There is no impact at all
b. The pain doesn't extend below the knees
c. The resistance and buoyancy protect and strengthen
d. Heaviness is the most common cause of back pain

4. The spinal column has three functions, two of which are:

a. Movement and assisting movement in other areas
b. Cushioning the body and protecting the body
c. Muscles and ligaments
d. Support of the body and protection of the spinal cord

(continued on next page)

5. The section of the spinal column that has the broadest and heaviest vertebrae is called:

a. The cervical region
b. The coccygeal region
c. The thoracic region
d. The lumbar region

6. The thoracic region of the spinal column is made up of:

a. 12 vertebrae with each connected to two ribs
b. 10 vertebrae with each connected to a rib
c. 12 vertebrae with 10 connected to a rib
d. 16 vertebrae with 12 connected to a rib

7. In regard to the spinal column, the rectus abdominus

a. protects the spinal cord
b. supports the spinal column from the front
c. keeps the disks from rubbing against each other
c. is the strongest support muscle for the spinal column

8. The following problem would exclude a person from a home program:

a. He has two hours per day with no pain
b. He has pain only in his back
c. He has pain only shooting down to his foot
d. He has had recurrent back problems in the past 6 months

9. The following person would qualify for a BackHab program

a. He has numbness in his toes
b. He was just in a car accident

c. He has boring pain in the low back
d. He also has bladder problems

10. The following is <u>not</u> a guideline for the BackHab program

a. The two hour pain rule applies
b. Cooler water is better for the joints
c. Pain means stop
d. Ideal water depth is midriff

Water Walking Log

Day / Week	S	M	T	W	T	F	S
1			Do the Thermal Warmup, Pre-Stretch, Cardio Warmup, Aerobic Groups 1 & 2, Cooldown, Toning, & Post Stretch		Repeat Tuesday's Workout		Read Chapter 9 for guide-lines
2			Do the Thermal Warmup, Pre-Stretch, Cardio Warmup, Aerobic Groups 1, 2 & 3, Cooldown, Toning, & Post Stretch		Repeat Tuesday's Workout		
3			Do the Thermal Warmup, Pre-Stretch, Cardio Warmup, Aerobic Groups 1, 2, 3 & 4, Cooldown, Toning, & Post Stretch		Repeat Tuesday's Workout		
4	Repeat Thursday's workout			Repeat Monday's workout		Repeat Monday's workout	Review Chapter 9 again
5		Do the same workout as week 4		Do the same workout as week 4		Do the same workout as week 4	
6		Do the Thermal Warmup, Pre-Stretch, Cardio Warmup, Aerobic Groups 1, 2, 3, 4 & 5, Cooldown, Toning, & Post Stretch		Repeat Monday's workout		Repeat Monday's workout	
7		Full Program		Full Program		Full Program	
8		Full Program		Full Program		Full Program	Full Program
9		Full Program		Full Program		Full Program	Full Program

Food Guide Pyramid

A Guide to Daily Food Choices

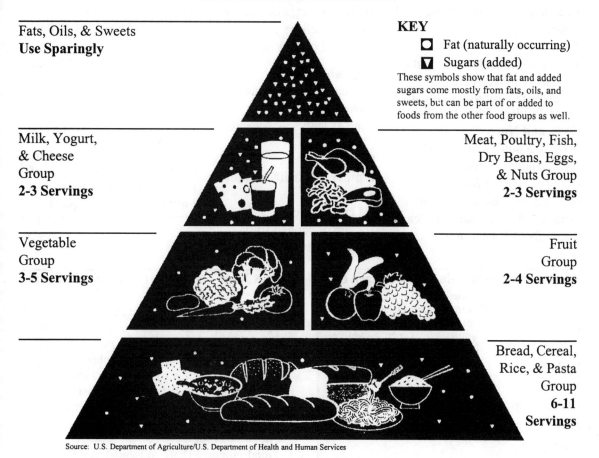

Fats, Oils, & Sweets
Use Sparingly

KEY
- ▢ Fat (naturally occurring)
- ▼ Sugars (added)

These symbols show that fat and added sugars come mostly from fats, oils, and sweets, but can be part of or added to foods from the other food groups as well.

Milk, Yogurt,
& Cheese
Group
2-3 Servings

Meat, Poultry, Fish,
Dry Beans, Eggs,
& Nuts Group
2-3 Servings

Vegetable
Group
3-5 Servings

Fruit
Group
2-4 Servings

Bread, Cereal,
Rice, & Pasta
Group
**6-11
Servings**

Source: U.S. Department of Agriculture/U.S. Department of Health and Human Services

Use the Food Guide Pyramid to help you eat better every day . . . the Dietary Guidelines way. Start with plenty of Breads, Cereals, Rice, and Pastas; Vegetables; and Fruits. Add two to three servings from the Milk group and two to three servings from the Meat group.

Each of these food groups provides some, but not all of the nutrients you need. No one food group is more important than another - for good health you need them all. Go easy on fats, oils, and sweets, the foods in the small tip of the Pyramid.

How to Use The Daily Food Guide

What counts as one serving?

Breads, Cereals, Rice, and Pasta
1 slice of bread
1/2 cup of cooked rice or pasta
1/2 cup of cooked cereal
1 ounce of ready-to-eat cereal

Meat, Poultry, Fish, Dry Beans, Eggs, and Nuts
2-1/2 to 3 ounces of cooked lean meat, poultry, or fish
Count 1/2 cup of cooked beans, or 1 egg, or 2 tablespoons of peanut butter as 1 ounce of lean meat (about 1/3 serving)

Milk, Yogurt, and Cheese
1 cup of milk or yogurt
1-1/2 to 2 ounces of cheese

Vegetables
1/2 cup of chopped raw or cooked vegetables
1 cup of leafy raw vegetables

Fruits
1 piece of fruit or melon wedge
3/4 cup of juice
1/2 cup of canned fruit
1/4 cup of dried fruit

Fats, Oils, and Sweets
LIMIT CALORIES FROM THESE
especially if you need to lose weight

> The amount you eat may be more than one serving. For example, a dinner portion of spaghetti would count as two or three servings of pasta.

How many servings do you need each day?

	Women & some older adults	Children, teen girls, active women, most men	Teen boys & active men
Calorie level*	about 1,600	about 2,200	about 2,800
Bread group	6	9	11
Vegetable group	3	4	5
Fruit group	2	3	4
Milk group	**2-3	**2-3	**2-3
Meat group	2, for a total of 5 ounces	2, for a total of 6 ounces	3 for a total of 7 ounces

*These are the calorie levels if you choose lowfat, lean foods from the 5 major food groups and use foods from the fats, oils, and sweets group sparingly.

**Women who are pregnant or breastfeeding, teenagers, and young adults to age 24 need 3 servings.

A Closer Look at Fat and Added Sugars

The small tip of the Pyramid shows fats, oils, and sweets. These are foods such as salad dressings, cream, butter, margarine, sugars, soft drinks, candies, and sweet desserts. Alcoholic beverages are also part of this group. These foods provide calories but few vitamins and minerals. Most people should go easy on foods from this group.

Some fat or sugar symbols are shown in the other food groups. That's to remind you that some foods in these groups can also be high in fat and added sugars, such as cheese or ice cream from the milk group, or french fries from the vegetable group. When choosing foods for a healthful diet, consider the fat and added sugars in your choices from all the food groups, not just fats, oils, and sweets from the Pyramid tip.

BackHab Class Forms

If you are teaching a BackHab class you may want to use these forms.

<u>MEDICAL CLEARANCE FORM</u>

INSTRUCTOR NAME: _____
ADDRESS: _____
PHONE NUMBER: _____
FACILITY: _____

Your patient, _____, has applied to participate in an aquatic
BackHab program. The class meets three times a week for one half hour and involves
walking forward, backward and sideways through the water and some edge-of-the-pool
exercises. For example:

  Isometric and concentric abdominal and oblique work
  Strength work for the gluteals, abductors and adductors
  Flexibility work for the iliopsoas and low back muscles

We will be doing movements that include slow and controlled spinal rotation, flexion and
lateral flexion. The work will all be in a moderate range of motion geared toward each
person's individual capabilities.

I am planning to administer the Kraus Weber back tests prior to the 8 week program, and
again after weeks 4 and 8.

This program is geared toward participants who have low back pain. It can be chronic back
pain or pain from recovering from back injury or surgery BUT they must be finished with
primary therapy, and have your release to attend.

The goal is lessened pain through better muscle balance, tone and endurance. This is not an
aerobic program. There is no cardiorespiratory component.

A guard will be on duty and another instructor and I will be with the participants during the entire program.

Please list any medications that your patient is currently taking and how they will affect the BackHab workout.

Medication and Effect:

_____

_____

_____

Please list any restrictions, modifications or recommendations for your patient's BackHab program.

_____

_____

Please list any special concerns you may have regarding this patient (i.e. arrhythmia, total hip, arthritis, etc.).

_____

_____

Sincerely,

. . . .

My patient, _____, has my approval to enroll in a BackHab program at the District Aquatic Center with the above restrictions, modifications and recommendations.

PHYSICIAN'S (THERAPIST'S) SIGNATURE_____

ADDRESS _____

PHONE NUMBER _____DATE_____

HEALTH HISTORY FORM

NAME _____SEX _____

ADDRESS _____

CITY _____ STATE_____ ZIP_____

PHONE NUMBER: home_____work_____

DATE OF BIRTH _____

TODAY'S DATE _____

PHYSICIAN'S NAME _____

   PHONE NUMBER _____

    ADDRESS_____

EMERGENCY CONTACT PERSON _____

   PHONE NUMBER: home_____work_____

   RELATIONSHIP_____

I have swimming abilities which would enable me to save my own life.   YES   NO
                                                        (circle one)

YES   NO

☐   ☐   1. Has your physician ever implied or said that you have heart disease or any heart trouble?

☐   ☐   2. Do you often have pains in your chest?

YES	NO	
☐	☐	1. Has your physician ever implied or said that you have heart disease or any heart trouble?
☐	☐	2. Do you often have pains in your chest?
☐	☐	3. Do you often feel faint or dizzy?
☐	☐	4. Are you sedentary and over 65?
☐	☐	5. Has your physician said that your blood pressure is too high?
☐	☐	6. Has your physician ever said you have any bone, joint or muscle problem that could be aggravated by exercise?
☐	☐	7. Is there any physical reason why you should not participate in any type of exercise?

Do you or have you ever had: (check all that apply)

☐   hypertension (high blood pressure)

☐   high blood lipids and cholesterol level

☐   smoking habits

☐   obesity (20 lbs or more overweight)

☐   family history of heart disease

☐   atherosclerosis (hardening of the arteries)

☐   diabetes

☐   excessive stress

☐   history of heart problems

☐   chronic illness

☐   advice from a physician not to exercise

☐   difficulty with physical exercise (dizziness, breathlessness, recent sur
     gery, pregnancy status, anxiety or depression)

☐   muscle, joint or back disorders

☐   history of lung problems

☐   asthma or other allergies

☐   arthritis or other joint problems

What is your current level of activity? (circle one)
        sedentary
        moderately active
        extremely active

List all medications you are currently taking and the frequency of use.

_____

_____

_____

_____

_____

_____

_____

_____

_____

_____

Student Pain Questionnaire

1. How bad is the pain on a scale from 1-10 with ten being excruciating?
    (circle one)   1   2   3   4   5   6   7   8   9   1 0

2. Where is the pain located? _____
    _____

3. What type of pain is it? (circle all that apply)
    Shooting
    Spasm
    Dull ache
    Stinging
    Throbbing

4. Do you have pain at night when you sleep? _____

5. What percent of the day (waking hours) or how often do you experience the following
    type of pain?
    Shooting   _____
    Spasm   _____
    Dull ache   _____
    Stinging   _____
    Throbbing   _____

6. How many hours each day do you spend
    Sitting?   _____
    Lying down?   _____
    Moving?   _____

7. Approximately how many times each day do you
    Reach up overhead?   _____
    Reach down to chair seat level?   _____
    Bend down to the floor?   _____

8. Do you participate in any type of exercise?_____

    What type?_____

    How often each week?_____

    How long each time?_____

    How vigorously?_____

STUDENT

NAME_____DATE_____

Representation, Release And Agreement
(PLEASE READ CAREFULLY AND SIGN BELOW)

"I, fully understanding that the programs and exercises of THE BACKHAB PROGRAM require moderate physical activity, hereby represent and acknowledge that my physical condition permits me to participate in THE BACKHAB programs and exercises. I further acknowledge that I have been advised that at any time I am having physical difficulty, I will immediately inform the Class Teacher and will be automatically excused from classes. I have volunteered to participate in this program and accept the responsibility. I understand that the possibility of exercise injuries or disorders does exist. I acknowledge and accept those risks.

I further realize that I will not be accepted for participation in the program if instructor knows of any reason why my participation would be dangerous to my health.

I also release and discharge on my behalf of myself, my heirs, assigns and successor in interest, all officers, directors, agents, and employees and other representatives of THE BACKHAB PROGRAM and its insurers, from any and all claim, damages, demands, and liabilities arising out of or in any way related to participation in THE BACKHAB PROGRAM activities and the use of any of its exercises, procedures or other results attained therefrom.

_____   _____
MEMBER'S SIGNATURE   DATE

BackHab Resources

Adolph Kiefer and Associates
       1700 Kiefer Drive
       Zion, IL 60099
       Phone: 800-323-4071
       Fax: 800-654-7946 / 847-746-8888
       Web Site: www.kiefer.com
Pool and aquatic program equipment. Call for a free catalog.

Ai Chi - Balance, Harmony and Healing
       Contact: Aquatic Exercise Association or Adolph Kiefer
This comprehensive, in-depth book takes experienced practitioners to a new level of Ai Chi
practice, yet will be useful to the novice as well. The book compares the traditional Ai Chi
program for an average healthy adult with modifications for special populations. Ai Chi Ne
(partner stretching) and Cultivating the Chi (advanced Ai Chi positions) are defined and illus-
trated.

American Heart Association
       7272 Greenville Ave.
       Dallas, TX 75231-4596
       Phone: 214-373-6300
       Web Site: www.americanheart.org
AHA produces and distributes print and audiovisual materials for health professionals and the
general public, answers inquiries, maintains a resource library and makes referrals to other
sources of information.

American National Red Cross
       8111 Gatehouse Road 6th Floor
       Falls Church, VA 22042
       Phone: 703-206-7625
       Fax: 703-206-7673
       Web Site: www.redcross.org
The Red Cross offers water safety programs throughout the country.

American Physical Therapy Association
        323 De La Mare Avenue
        Fairhope, AL 36532
        Phone: 334-990-5713
        Fax: 334-990-8019

American Public Health Association
        1015 15th Street NW Suite 300
        Washington, DC 20005
        Phone: 202-789-5611
Disseminates general knowledge on health issues.

Arthritis Foundation, National Office
        1330 West Peachtree Street
        Atlanta, GA 30309
        Phone: 404-872-7100
        Web Site: www.arthritis.org
Distributes information and educates about arthritis.

Aquatic Access, Inc.
        417 Dorsey Way
        Louisville, KY 40223
        Phone: 800-325-LIFT/502-425-5817
        Fax: 502-425-9607
        Web Site: www.aquaticaccess.com
Aquatic Access manufactures water power lifts for easy entry into the pool.

Aquatic Exercise Association
        3439 Technology Drive Suite 6
        Nokomis, FL 34275
        Phone: 888-AEA-WAVE
        Fax: 941-486-8820
        Web Site: www.aeawave.com
AEA is an international clearinghouse of information with a bimonthly newsletter and a selection

of aquatic books, audio cassettes, and videos. They also offer the universal teacher certification program and other educational conferences and programs. The AEA's newsletter, AKWA Letter; is available by subscription.

Aquatic Therapy & Rehab Institute, Inc.
    45450 Cottage Row
    Chassell, MI 49916
    Phone: 906-482-9500
    Fax: 906-482-4388
    Web Site: www.arti.org
ATRI offers international symposiums, certifications and memberships for medical professionals.

Aquatics International Magazine
    4160 Wilshire Blvd.
    Los Angeles, CA 90010
    Phone: 323-964-4800
    Fax: 323-964-4842
    Web Site: www.aquaticsintl@earthlink.com

AQUATICS - The Complete Reference Guide for Aquatic Fitness Professionals by Ruth Sova
    Contact: Aquatic Exercise Association or Adolph Kiefer and Associates.
This book is an encyclopedia of aquatic fitness information for professionals. It is the only book available covering both the complete spectrum of the aquatic fitness industry and peripheral disciplines affecting it. AQUATICS covers all the information needed by the aquatic professional to begin a safe, effective, successful aquatic program.

Consumer Information Center
    Dept. 314-A
    Pueblo, CO 81009
    Phone: 719-948-3334
The 1990 Dietary Guidelines recommend a varied and balanced diet. Suggested daily fruit consumption is 2-4 servings, and suggested vegetable consumption is 3-5 servings a day. Obtain 1-10 free copies by writing to the above address. Ask for Nutrition and Your Health: ietary Guidelines for Americans, Third Edition, 1990, Home and Garden Bulletin No. 232.

Country Technology, Inc.
        P. O. Box 87
        Gays Mills, WI 54631
        Phone: 608-735-4718
        Fax: 608-735-4859
        Email: ctech@mwt.net
Vital Signs, a catalog of products for rehabilitation, sports medicine, and physical fitness, is
available from Country Technology.

Fitness First Products
        P. O. Box 251
        Shawnee Mission, KS 66201
        Phone: 800-421-1791
        Fax: 800-421-0036
        Web site: www.fitness1st.com

Fitness Swimmer Magazine
        c/o Rodale Publications
        33R East Moinor Street
        Emmaus, PA 18098
        Phone: 800-846-0086 / 610-867-8939
        Fax: 610-967-9131
        Web Site: www.fitnessswimmer.com

Fitness Wholesale
        895-A Hampshire Road
        Stow, OH 44224
        Phone: 800-537-5512
Fitness Wholesale carries numerous products for use in aquatic exercise and therapy. Call
for a free catalog.

HydroFit
    1328 W. Second Avenue
    Eugene, OR 97401
    Phone: 800-346-7295 / 541-484-4361
    Fax: 541-484-1443
    Web Site: www,hydrofit.com
Makers of aquatic fitness gear. Call for free catalog.

Hydro-Tone Fitness Systems
    16691 Gothard Street, Suite M
    Huntington Beach, CA 92647
    Phone: 800-622-8663 / 714-848-8284
    Fax: 714-848-9035
    Web Site: www.hydrotone.com
Aquatic exercise and therapy equipment.

National Health Information Clearinghouse
    P. O. Box 1133
    Washington, DC 20013-1133
    Phone: 800-336-4797
Answers consumer and health professional's inquiries, operates telephone "hotline"
service, produces and distributes print materials for professionals as well as the general
public. Develops conputerized databases, maintains a resourse library, makes referrals to other
sources of information, and provides reference services.

OPTP
    3700 Annapolis Lane, Suite 175
    Minneapolis, MN 55447
    Phone: 800-367-7393 / 612-553-0452
    Fax: 612-553-9355
    Web Site: www.optp.com
Orthopedic physical therapy products, professional health care products, resistive exercise
products, bands, videos, and books.

Recreonics, Inc.
    7696 Zionsville Road
    Indianapolis, IN 46268

    Phone: 800-428-3254 / 502-456-5706
    Fax: 502-458-9777
    Web Site: www.recreonics.com
    Email: aquatics@recreonics.com
Pool and aquatic program equipment. Call for a free catalog.

Sprint/Rothhammer International, Inc.
    P. O. Box 3840
    San Luis Obispo, CA 93403-3840
    Phone: 800-235-2156
    Fax: 800-652-6364 / 805-541-5339
    Web Site: www.sprintaquatics.com
Sprint/Rothhammer offers numerous water-related products.

YMCA of the U.S.A.
    101 N. Wacker Drive
    Chicago, IL 60606
    Phone: 800-USA-YMCA

YWCA of the U.S.A.
    726 Broadway
    New York, NY 10003
    Phone: 212-614-2700

Pool Polices

You should know the following types of information about your pool.

The policies of the aquatic center are enforced to maintain the health and safety of all patrons. Please follow these policies.

1. No food, alcohol, gum or tobacco are permitted. There is no smoking allowed in the facility and participants under the influence of alcohol will be asked to leave.

2. No glass of any kind is permitted in the pool area.

3. No running in the hallways, stairs, locker rooms or pool area is permitted.

4. No pets are allowed.

5. All forms of jewelry should be removed before entering the pool. It is the exerciser's responsibility to secure all valuables.

6. Swimsuits or appropriate aquatic exercise wear must be worn by all exercisers. Cut offs or other clothes with lose threads are not permitted.

7. Exercisers must shower before entering the pool.

8. Exercisers with skin infections, open sores or rashes are not permitted to use the pool.

9. Conduct that may endanger the welfare and comfort of others is prohibited.

10. In case of fire alarm: Participants in the pool should use the double exit doors on the west side of the pool. Participants in the locker rooms should exit through the south doors via the hallway.

11. In case of tornado and civil defense evacuation: Participants in the pool should move to the middle school locker room. Participants in the locker rooms should stay in the locker room.

12. In case of a pool emergency: Exit the pool and wait on the benches until class is resumed or canceled.

13. If you currently take medications which may be required during exercise, please keep them at the pool edge and explain the symptoms and administration of the medication to the instructor.

Bibliography

Bates, Andrea and Hanson, Norm. Aquatic Exercise Therapy.

Bates, Larry. P.T. "Examine Your Back," S.W.E.A.T. August, 1992, pg. 18.

Bejeck, Bill, CSCS, CCS. "All About Abs," IDEA Health and Fitness Source, (March 2000). Pp. 29-33.

Boden SD, Davis DO, Dina TS. "Abnormal magnetic-resonance scans of the lumbar spine in asymptomatic subjects: a prospective investigation." J Bone Joint Surg Am 1990;72(3):403-408.

Bohannon, R.W., P.T. "Stretching for Low Back Pain," Physical Therapy Forum, August 5, 1992, pg. 10.

Bronner S, Brownstein B. The organization of movement of the joints of the lower limb and trunk during a skilled ballet technique. Submitted for publication.

Brooks, Douglas, MS, and Candice Copeland-Brooks. "Uncovering The Myths of Abdominal Exercise," IDEA Today, (April 1993), pp. 42-49.

Bundschuh, Lauren. Creating Positive Verbal Responses Lecture.

Burdendo, Igor and Connors, Edmund. An American-Russian Approach to Fitness and Health.

Carey, Anthony, MA, CSCS. "Building Functional Fitness," IDEA Personal Trainer, (March 1998), pp. 21-27.

Cheatle M.D., Esterhai J.L. "Pelvic traction as treatment for acute back pain:efficacious, benign, or deleterious," Spine, 16(12), 1379-1381. 1991.

Chek, Paul, MSS, HHP, NMT. "Suspension System for The Spine," Massage & Bodywork, (December/January 1999), pp. 55-58.

Chossek, and C. Mathies. Back In Shape. Port Washington, Wisconsin: Dance Slimnastics, 1985.

Cirullo, Judy. "Part I: Attaining and Maintaining a Healthy Back Through Wise Water Work," The AKWA Letter, Vol. 3, No. 1 (May, 1989) p. 1.

Cirullo, Judy. "Part II: Attaining and Maintaining a Healthy Back Through Wise Water Work," The AKWA Letter, Vol. 3, No. 2 (July, 1989), pp. 5-6.

Clippinger-Robertson, Karen, M.S.P.E. "Reducing the Risks of Forward Flexion," IDEA Today, May, 1991.

Cole, Andrew J, MD, Eagleston, Richard E., PT, ATC, Moschetti, Marilou, BS,PTA, Sinnett, Edward, BAS, "Spine Pain:Aquatic Rehabilitation Strategies," Back and Musculoskeletal Rehabilitation, (October, 1994), pp. 273-286.

Cypress, B.K. "Characteristics of Physician Visits For Back Symptoms: A National Perspective", American Journal Public Health, 73: 389-395, 1983.

Darragh, Angela, PT. "Training Clients and Spinal Post," IDEA Personal Trainer, (May 1999), pp. 42-51.

DeMond, T.E. "Getting Back in Shape", American Fitness, July/August 1992, pg.41-42.

DeTroyer A, Estenne M, Ninane V, et al. "Transersus abdominis muscle function in humans," J Appl Physiol 68:1010-1016, 1990.

Diffendal, Jill. "Living with Spina Bifida," advance for Occupational Therapy Practitioners, (February 19, 2001), pp. 10, 27.

Edlin, and E. Golanty. Health and Wellness: A Holistic Approach. Boston, Massachusetts: Jones and Bartlett Publishers, 1992.

Friedman P, Eisen G. The Pilates Method of Physical and Mental Conditioning. Doubleday, New York, 1980.

Frymoyer JW, Gordon SL. "New Perspectives on Low Back Pain". Park Ridge, IL: American Academy of Orthopaedic Surgeons: 1989:4-8, 215-241.

Gaines, MaryBeth Pappas. "Aqua Abdominal Techniques Produce Firm Results," AKWA letter, November, 1990.

Genuario, Susan E., and Joseph J. Vegso. "The Use of Swimming Pool in the Rehabilitation and Reconditioning of Athletic Injuries," Contemporary Orthopedics, Vol. 20, No. 4 (April, 1990) pp. 381-387.

Geraidy, Bafra, Sarmidy, Sana. "A Muscular Endurance Training Program for Symmetrical and Asymmetrical Manual Lifting Tasks," Journal of Occupational Medicine, January 1990; 32 (3): 226-233.

Grabiner M, Koh T, Ghazawi AE. "Decoupling of bilateral parspinal excitation in subjects with low back pain," Spine 17:1219-1223, 1992.

Harrison R., Bulstrode S. "Percentage Weight-bearing during Partia Iimmersion in the Hydrotherapy Pool". Physiotherapy Practice, 60-63, 1987.

Hides J, Stokes M, Saide M, et al. "Evidence of lumbar multifidus wasting ipsilateral to symptoms in patients with acute/subacute low back pain," Spine 19:165-172, 1994.

Hodges PW, Richardson CA. "Contraction of the abdominal muscles associated with movement of the lower limb," Physical Therapy 77:132-144, 1997.

Hodges P, Richardson CA. "Inefficient muscular stabilization of the lumbar spine associated with low back pain: a motor control evaluation of the transvesus abdominus," Spine 21:357-364, 1996.

Hughes, Daniel, MS, PT. "Aquatic Therapy in the Management of Low Back Dysfunction," Sports Medicine, Vol.7 No.2 (Summer 1992), pp. 10-15.

Imrie, David with Colleen Dimson. Goodbye Backache. New York: Avco Publishing, Inc. 1983.

Kemper, McIntosh, and T.M. Roberts. Healthwise Handbook: A Self-Care Manual For You. Boise, Idaho: Healthwise Incorporated, Ninth Edition, 1991.

Kendall, F. P., PT. Muscles Testing & Function.

Kibler WB. "Role of the scapula in overhead throwing motions," Contemporary Orthopedics 22:526-532, 1991.

Koury, Joanne. Aquatic Therapy Programming: Guidelines for Orthopedic Rehabilitation
Meyer, Ruth. H2ORx : Exercise Therapy Consultants and Aquatic Therapy Resources.

LaForge, Ralph. "Oh, My Aching Back," Executive Health Report, Oct. 1990, p. 6.

Levin S. "Aquatic Therapy: A Splashing Success for Arthritis and Injury Rehabilitation," Phys Sports Med, 19(10), 119-126, 1991.

Lopez-Antunez, L., MD. Atlas of Human Anatomy.

Luttgens, and Wells. Kinesiology—Scientific Basis of Human Motion. Seventh ed. W.B. Saunders College Publishing.

Massion J. Movement, posture, and equilibrium: interaction and coordination. Progress in Neurobiology 38:35-56, 1992.

Mayer, Gatchel, Mayer, et al. "A Prospective Two Year Study of Functional Restoration in Industrial Low Back Injury", JAMA, 1987; 258 (13); 1763-1767.

McElligott, Miscovich, Fielding, L.P. "Low Back Injury in Industry: The Value of a Recovery Program", Connecticut Medicine, 1989; 53:12: 711-715.

Melleby, Alexander. The Y's Way to a Healthy Back, National Director of the YMCA Health Back Program. New Century Publishers, Inc. 1982

Michel, Lane, Bjorkengren, et al. "Running and Lumbar Bone Density: A 5-Year Longitudinal Study," J Bone Miner Res, 1991, 6 (suppl 1), pg. 105

Miller MI, Medeiros JM. "Recruitment of internal oblique and transversus abdominis muscles during the eccentric phase of the curl-up exercise," Physical Therapy 67:1213-1217, 1987.

Milwaukee Public Schools. The Halliwick Method: Water Freedom for the Handicapped.

Mitchell, Terri. "The Use of Props in Water Exercise for Muscle Conditioning," The AKWA Letter, Vol. 3, No. 1(May, 1989) p. 6.

Moschetti, Marilou. Aquaphysics Made Simple, 1990, AquaTechnics, California.

Munnings, Frances. "Osteoporosis: What Is the Role of Exercise?", The Physician and SportsMedicine, Vol. 20, No. 6, June, 1992, pg. 127-138.

Nasher LM, McCollum G. "The organization of human postural mechanics: a formal basis and experimental synthesis," Behav Brain Sci 8:135-172. 1985.

Norkin CC, Levangie PK. Joint Structure and Function: A Comprehensive Review. Philadelphia, PA: F.A. Davis Co.: 1992:151-162.

Nottingham, Suzanne. "Training for Proprioiception & Function," Fitness Management, (February 2001), pp. 28-29.

O'Sullivan PB, Twomey L, Allison GT. "Dysfunction of the neuro-muscular system in the presence of low back pain – implications for physical therapy management." The Journal of Manual Manipulation Therapy 5:20-26, 1997.

Phillips, Greg. "Has the Bend Been Banned?" Aerobics and Fitness, January/February 1992.

PhysicalMind (R) Institute, 1807 Second Street #28/29, Santa Fe, NM 87505, 800-505-1990 Ruoti, Richard. Aquatic Therapy.

Physician and Sports Medicine: "Joe Montana: Back Exercises for a Super Bowl Winner," Phys Sports Med, 17(9), 188, 1989.

Putnam CA. Sequential motions of body segments during striking and throwing skills: descriptions and explanations. Journal of Biomechanics 26 (supplement 1): 125-135, 1993.

Rossignol, Suissa, Abernheim, L. "Working Disability Due To Occupational Back Pain: Three Year Follow-Up of 2,300 Compensated Workers in Quebec", Journal of Occupational Medicine, June 1988; 30: 6; 502-505.

Rowe, M.C. Backache At Work. Fairport, New York: Perinton Press, 1983.

Schatz, Mary Pullig. "Walk Your Back to Health," The Physician and Sportsmedicine, Vol 19, No. 5 (May, 1991) p. 127-128.

Scovazzo ML, Browne A, Pink M et al. "The painful shoulder during freestyle swimming. An electromyographic and cinematographic analysis of twelve muscles," American Journal of Sports Medicine 19:577-582, 1991.

Schrepfer, Robert W. and Julie Fritz. "A Comparison of Change in Visual Analogue Pain Rating of Acute Low Back Pain Patients Following Deep Water Walking or Deep Water Hanging," The Journal of Aquatic Physical Therapy, Vol. 8 No. 2 (Fall 2000), pp. 25-28.

Skinner, Alison and Thomson, Ann. Duffield's Exercise in Water.

Snook, S.H. "Approaches To The Control of Back Pain In Industry: Job Design, Job Placement and Education Training", State Art Rev Occupational Medicine, 1988; 3: 45-59.

Snook, S.H. "The Costs of Back Pain In Industry", Spine - State of the Art Review, 1987; 2: 1-5.

Sova, Ruth. AQUATICS: The Complete Reference Guide for Aquatic Fitness Professionals. Boston: Jones and Bartlett, 1991.

Spodnik, and Cogan, D.P. The 35-Plus Good Health Guide For Women. New York: Harper and Row, 1989.

Synergy Systems (R), 201 4th Street, Suite #322, Del Mar, CA 92014 (619) 792-5675

U.S. Department of Health and Human Services: Work Practices Guide of Manual Lifting. Washington D.C. Dhhs (Niosh) Pub. No. 81-122, 1981.

Vogel, Amanda, M.A. "Core Conditioning Takes Center Stage," IDEA Health & Fitness Source, (March 2001), pp. 32-38.

Vogel, Amanda, M.A. "Helping Clients Find Neutral Spine," ACE Certified News, pp. 6-7.

Walters, Peter H., PhD., CSCS. "Back to the Basics – Strengthening the Neglected Lower Back," ACSM's Health & Fitness Journal, (July/August 2000), pp. 19-25.

Webster, B.S., Snook, S. "The Cost of Compensable Low Back Pain", Journal of Occupational Medicine, January 1990, 32(1): 13-15.

Wescott, Wayne L. "Low Back Insurance," Power Source, Vol. 1, Number 1 (Winter 1992), pp. 6-7.

Wohfahrt D, Jull G, Richardson C. "The relationship between the dynamic and static function of abdominal muscles," Australian Physiotherapy 39:9-13, 1993.

Yoke, Mary, M.A. "The Low Back Low Down: Pain Prevention," American Fitness, (July/ August 2000), pp. 47-56.